Healthcare Activism

Healthcare Activism

Markets, Morals, and the Collective Good

Edited by
SUSI GEIGER

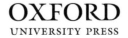

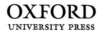

Great Clarendon Street, Oxford, OX2 6DP,
United Kingdom

Oxford University Press is a department of the University of Oxford.
It furthers the University's objective of excellence in research, scholarship,
and education by publishing worldwide. Oxford is a registered trade mark of
Oxford University Press in the UK and in certain other countries

© the several contributors 2021

The moral rights of the authors have been asserted

First Edition published in 2021

Impression: 1

All rights reserved. No part of this publication may be reproduced, stored in
a retrieval system, or transmitted, in any form or by any means, without the
prior permission in writing of Oxford University Press, or as expressly permitted
by law, by licence or under terms agreed with the appropriate reprographics
rights organization. Enquiries concerning reproduction outside the scope of the
above should be sent to the Rights Department, Oxford University Press, at the
address above

You must not circulate this work in any other form
and you must impose this same condition on any acquirer

Published in the United States of America by Oxford University Press
198 Madison Avenue, New York, NY 10016, United States of America

British Library Cataloguing in Publication Data

Data available

Library of Congress Control Number: 2021938260

ISBN 978–0–19–886522–3

DOI: 10.1093/oso/9780198865223.001.0001

Printed and bound by
CPI Group (UK) Ltd, Croydon, CR0 4YY

Links to third party websites are provided by Oxford in good faith and
for information only. Oxford disclaims any responsibility for the materials
contained in any third party website referenced in this work.

Preface

This book was conceived and individual contributions first discussed during a workshop entitled "Health Activism between Markets and Morals" on September 20, 2019 in Dublin, organized and funded through the ERC MISFIRES project (grant agreement no. 771217).[1] Its context of completion however, just over eighteen months later, could not have been more different, especially for a volume that takes healthcare as its central concern. As this volume goes to print, over 175 million people have contracted the SARS Covid 2 coronavirus and tragically over 3.8 million lives have been lost globally. In addition, the pandemic has occasioned a panoply of political reactions, many of which are unprecedented in modern times in their scope and impact on individual and collective freedoms. Within the span of a year, the virus has changed fundamentally how many of us live, work, learn, and interact—and it has also fundamentally and perhaps forever changed the value we attribute to public health, healthcare security, pharmaceutical innovation, and the collective good in healthcare. Relevant to this volume, the virus has also influenced which voices are heard and which are silenced in public health decision making.

While a volume on healthcare activism can evidently not ignore the current events, its individual chapters had been prepared before the virus hit the globe, and in discussions with authors and author teams we agreed to keep the integrity of the chapters and their place in the book's structure intact—that is, not to pivot from their substantive subject matter to the ubiquitous Covid-19 topic. Instead, Chapter 1 takes on the task of both introducing the reader to some of the conceptual and empirical issues the volume grapples with beyond the current dynamics as well as contextualizing these through the Covid-19 pandemic. In some instances, this is a relatively easy undertaking, as the pandemic crystallizes and catalyzes some of the chapters' core messages—for instance when reflecting on governments' rapid rollout of Covid-19 tracker apps, which echoes some of the issues on the role of "datafication" in contemporary healthcare and the "ruinations and repairs" this process causes that Hoeyer and Langstrup cover in Chapter 5. In other instances, the pandemic acts as a counterintuitive, particularly in the question of why some of the activists and civil society voices that we may have expected to come to the fore during the pandemic are so relatively muted—there was, for instance, a relatively silent acquiescence of the "cocooning" strategy meant to protect the over 70s in countries such as the United Kingdom and Ireland by age action associations.

It is important to situate the current volume's authors' and editor's perspectives: we are speaking from positions within academia in the Global North. While the geographic contexts of the book's empirical chapters range from the welfare states of Sweden and Denmark (Lindén and Hoeyer/Langstrup) through the arguably more marketized healthcare landscapes of Ireland and the United Kingdom (Moran/Mountford and Cheded/Hopkinson), to the contentious multi-payer system of the United States (Gottlieb), the book rests with an avowedly partial perspective of healthcare activism. Large parts of the globe, their concerns, public debates, and their unique forms of activism are absent from this current volume. Though a broader global perspective undoubtedly would have been desirable, thematic cohesion and comparability of cases would have suffered as a consequence. The contours of a fully global form of healthcare activism is just crystallizing at the moment as the pandemic shows good health and wellbeing to be a truly global public good. However, working thoroughly through such a global perspective on healthcare activism remains the task for a future volume.

If such a future volume ever comes to be, it is purely courtesy of those who have helped me make this one a reality even in the strangest of circumstances. First and foremost, these are of course the book contributors and the presenters at the ERC MISFIRES workshop in Dublin in 2019, who have not only stimulated a lot of my thinking through their own research and through the many debates we have enjoyed, but also through sharing many of my concerns about the marketization of contemporary healthcare systems. Friends and colleagues who have acted as reviewers for this volume have greatly helped enhance its logic and value—thank you! A huge thanks also goes to my MISFIRES project team for many stimulating discussions: Gemma Watts, Emma Stendahl, Ilaria Galasso, Stephen Nicola, Théo Bourgeron, Sula Awad, Fernardos Ongolly Kredgie, and Simeon Vidolov. My former PhD student, friend, and colleague Nicola Mountford has accompanied me throughout my now decade-long journey into the weird and wonderful universe that is healthcare. And my friends at Access to Medicines Ireland have accepted me into the world of healthcare activism proper and showed me the ropes. I owe thanks to the people at Oxford University Press who bought into this volume's vision and helped it to be realized, in particular Adam Swallow and Jenny King. Most importantly, of course, Gerry, Killian, Clara, and Maia—I would be nothing without you guys.

Note

1. The multidisciplinary project "MISFIRES and Market Innovation", or MISFIRES for short, started in August 2018 and is an EU H2020 European Research Council project on market contests and innovation in healthcare. The aim of the project is to make healthcare markets more participatory and to innovate together for better markets. I gratefully acknowledge the funding received from the European Research Council under the European Union's Horizon 2020 research and innovation program (grant agreement No. 771217), which has funded the workshop that the volume is based on as well as my own and Ilaria Galasso's contributions to this volume.

Contents

List of Figures and Tables	xi
List of Contributors	xiii

1. Healthcare Activism, Marketization, and the Collective Good   1
   Susi Geiger

2. Preventing "Exit," Eliciting "Voice": Patient, Participant,
   and Public Involvement as Invited Activism in Precision
   Medicine and Genomics Initiatives   28
   Ilaria Galasso and Susi Geiger

3. War on Diseases: Patient Organizations' Problematization
   and Exploration of Market Issues   55
   Vololona Rabeharisoa and Liliana Doganova

4. "Please Don't Put a Price on Our Lives": Social Media and the
   Contestation of Value in Ireland's Pricing of Orphan Drugs   86
   Gillian Moran and Nicola Mountford

5. Datafying the Patient Voice: The Making of Pervasive
   Infrastructures as Processes of Promise, Ruination, and Repair   116
   Klaus Hoeyer and Henriette Langstrup

6. Initiators, Controllers, and Influencers: Enacting Patient
   Advocacy Roles in Cervical Cancer Screening Policy Practices   140
   Lisa Lindén

7. Heroes, Villains, and Victims: Tracing Breast Cancer
   Activist Movements   165
   Mohammed Cheded and Gillian Hopkinson

8. The Fantastical Empowered Patient   198
   Samantha D. Gottlieb

9. Markets, Morals, and the Collective Good after Covid-19   224
   Barbara Prainsack and Hendrik Wagenaar

Index   237

List of Figures and Tables

Figures

4.1. Tweet categories by @YesOrkambi	94
4.2. Tweet categories by @SMAIrelandCom	95
4.3. The assessment process for drug reimbursement in Ireland	95
4.4. Timeline of key YesOrkambi campaign highlights	98
4.5. Timeline of key political actions highlighted by YesOrkambi	100
4.6. Timeline of key SpinrazaNow campaign and political highlights	102
4.7. Comparison of tweet categories	104
4.8. The roles and impact of social media within healthcare	109

Tables

7.1. Summary of the dramatis personae featured in the social movement narratives analyzed	187

List of Contributors

Mohammed Cheded is Lecturer at Lancaster University Management School. He is primarily interested in the sociological aspects of consumption, markets, and health. His research takes an interdisciplinary perspective drawing on sociology, anthropology, and linguistics, focusing on topics such as inequality, identity construction, and power relations.

Liliana Doganova is Associate Professor at the Centre de sociologie de l'innovation, Mines-ParisTech, PSL University. At the intersection of economic sociology and science and technology studies, her work has focused on business models, the valorization of public research, and markets for bio- and clean technologies. She has published in journals such as *Economy and Society*, the *Journal of Cultural Economy*, *Research Policy*, and *Science and Public Policy*. She is the author of *Valoriser la science* (2013) and co-author of *Capitalization: A Cultural Guide* (2017).

Ilaria Galasso is a postdoctoral researcher in the ERC MISFIRES project at University College Dublin. She has a background in ethical and political philosophy and philosophy of science and a PhD in science and technology studies. Her work focuses on social and health equity in the context of precision medicine. Her current research explores practices of public and patient involvement in genomics research as strategies to understand and meet the interests and needs of all social groups, including minorities and underserved populations.

Susi Geiger is Full Professor of Marketing and Market Studies in the College of Business, University College Dublin, and holder of a European Research Council Consolidator Grant, "MISFIRES and Market Innovation," which studies activism in healthcare markets. Her research focuses on how complex markets are organized, with specific interests in digital and healthcare markets in the context of social justice concerns. She has published numerous journal articles on these issues and co-edited the volume *Concerned Markets* (2014). Susi is also a member of Access to Medicines Ireland, a non-profit group campaigning for equitable access to medicines and medical technologies.

Samantha D. Gottlieb is a medical anthropologist who explores the complexities of healthcare and technologies, both material and digital. She focuses on patient activisms and advocacy through the lens of the larger health ecosystem in which people must navigate. She has worked in academia and private industry. She is currently a user experience researcher at Fitbit, which was acquired by Google, Inc., during the publishing process of this chapter.

xiv   LIST OF CONTRIBUTORS

Klaus Hoeyer is Professor at the Centre for Medical Science and Technology Studies, Department of Public Health, University of Copenhagen. His interests lie in the organization and regulation of the healthcare system, in particular with respect to the introduction of new medical technologies. His current research focuses on the drivers for and implications of intensified data sourcing in healthcare.

Gillian Hopkinson is Head of the Marketing Department at Lancaster University Management School. She is interested in marketing channels, particularly in food provision, access, and controversies. Focal empirical areas are questions of nutrition including sugar and genetically modified foods. Her work has been published in a wide variety of outlets including *Human Relations, Marketing Theory*, and *Industrial Marketing Management*.

Henriette Langstrup is Associate Professor at the Centre for Medical Science and Technology Studies, Department of Public Health, University of Copenhagen. Her research seeks to understand the social and organizational implications of technologies and arrangements aiming at improving clinical work and treatment through patient involvement and self-care.

Lisa Lindén holds a PhD in technology and social change and is a researcher at the Department of Sociology and Work Science, University of Gothenburg. Her work is focused on care and medicine, often with a focus on reproduction and sexual practices. In current projects she investigates gynecological cancer patient activism, the introduction of HPV vaccination for boys in Sweden, and former patients' experiences of gender confirmation treatment. She has published work in journals such as *Science, Technology and Human Values* and *Qualitative Research*, and in the edited volume *Gendering Drugs: Feminist Perspectives of Pharmaceuticals* (2017).

Gillian Moran is Assistant Professor in the School of Business at Maynooth University. Her research focuses on communications and influence in social media from different perspectives, such as business-to-consumer, consumer-to-consumer, and consumer-to-business. Gillian's research to date has been published in international peer-reviewed journals including the *Journal of Advertising Research, the Journal of Product and Brand Management*, and the *Journal of Marketing Communications*. Gillian also contributes articles to national media.

Nicola Mountford is Assistant Professor at Maynooth University's School of Business. Nicola's research interest is in how governments and other market actors can together find an optimum balance between the efficiency of a market and the social responsibilities of a state. Nicola held a Fulbright TechImpact Scholar Award in 2016–17 in the area of e-health and has published papers in journals such as *Organization Studies, Journal of Business Research*, the *International Journal of Integrated Care, Journal of Medical Internet Research*, and *Studies in Higher Education*.

Barbara Prainsack is Professor and Head of Department at the Department of Political Science at the University of Vienna, where she directs the Centre for the Study of

Contemporary Solidarity and the newly founded research platform "Governance of Digital Practices." Her work explores the social, regulatory, and ethical dimensions of biomedicine and bioscience, with current research projects focusing on personalized and "precision" medicine, on citizen participation in science and medicine, and the role of solidarity in medicine and healthcare. Barbara is also a member of the Austrian National Bioethics Committee advising the federal government in Vienna and of the European Group on Ethics in Science and New Technologies advising the European Commission.

Vololona Rabeharisoa is Professor at the Centre de sociologie de l'innovation, Mines-ParisTech, PSL University. She is interested in the increasing involvement of civil society organizations in scientific and technical activities. She studies the transformative effects of this involvement on the modes of production and dissemination of knowledge and on the forms of collective mobilization. She is investigating the engagement of patients' organizations with biomedical research, the governance of health, and the development of drugs and therapeutic strategies, notably in the area of rare diseases.

Hendrik Wagenaar (https://hendrikwagenaar.com) is Senior Academic Advisor to the International School for Government at King's College London, Fellow at the Institute for Advanced Studies in Vienna, and Adjunct Professor at the University of Canberra. He publishes in the areas of participatory democracy, interpretive policy analysis, deliberative policy analysis, prostitution policy, and practice theory. He is author of *Meaning in Action: Interpretation and Dialogue in Policy Analysis* (2011) and editor of *Deliberative Policy Analysis* (2003, with M. Hajer). In the area of prostitution research he published *Designing Prostitution Policy: Intention and Reality in Regulating the Sex Trade* (with Helga Amesberger and Sietske Altink, 2017).

1

Healthcare Activism, Marketization, and the Collective Good

Susi Geiger

In this introductory chapter I aim to define and connect the different component parts of this book's title: healthcare activism, markets, morals, and the collective good. I will argue that the way activists define and defend what they perceive as the collective good can only fully be understood by grasping how this good is shaped by other, often more dominant, stakeholders in healthcare: governmental institutions, professional experts, scientists, and private industry—the latter being a focal point of concern for this current volume. The central question that this book, across its individual chapters, asks is as follows: What is the role of civil society and activists in defining and defending the collective good in healthcare, especially in cases where that good is heavily shaped by market dynamics? It is a question that may never be answerable in full—as we will see in this chapter, even trying to define the public, common, or collective good is a slippery undertaking, and the answer to this question will always depend on the specific perspectives of those who embark on this definitional work. Likewise, tracing the activities of those who set out to advocate for it is likely to lead researchers into very diverse places that are often difficult to compare. Yet, this question has rarely been more pressing to pose than after a year where the world as most of us knew it was stopped in its tracks by a single, highly contagious, and often lethal virus. This virus has forced each country on the planet to reconsider the distribution of rights and responsibilities of their governments, companies, and citizens in relation to public and individual health. It has also reopened societal debates around what is "moral" or "right" for individual groups and society at large. The pandemic has in many places triggered calls for solidarity, a focus on community, and individual sacrifices for the good of society. At the same time, it has also highlighted the extent to which we have entrusted our collective welfare into the hands of a small number of often profit-driven firms.

Susi Geiger, *Healthcare Activism, Marketization, and the Collective Good* In: *Healthcare Activism: Markets, Morals, and the Collective Good.* Edited by: Susi Geiger, Oxford University Press. © Susi Geiger 2021.
DOI: 10.1093/oso/9780198865223.003.0001

1. Healthcare and Its Markets

One of the core propositions of this volume is that how healthcare activists define and defend the collective good is often in response to the role that the market as an institution and as an overarching logic (or way of thinking) has come to play in contemporary healthcare. This focus on the market may require some explanation, as for many, especially those of us living in countries with a universal healthcare system, the notion of the market does not sit naturally with healthcare. It may sit even less comfortably with healthcare *activism*, which tends to be directed at governments rather than private industry. For the purpose of this book I define healthcare activism as *political and pragmatic action aimed at criticizing and/or achieving change in the status quo of research, practice, and market structures in the healthcare domain*.

Of course, most of us are aware that behind any medical product or service, even if delivered and paid for through public bodies, there is "a market"—there's buying and selling; price-setting; negotiations and procurement; supply chains, research and development (R&D); and manufacturing. The market behind healthcare becomes apparent particularly in moments of breakdown, as for instance when manufacturers were unable to respond to the dramatically increased demand for personal and protective equipment for healthcare workers in the early stages of the Covid-19 pandemic. It became visible when certain medical supply chains were disrupted and patients left without vital medication; and it became a focal point of concern during the long wait for a Covid-19 vaccination, when certain nations negotiated advance purchase agreements of promising medications with pharmaceutical firms, threatening shortages in other regions (Matthews 2020). Yet, despite these apparent market breakdowns, the pharmaceutical industry was often portrayed as the only potential savior that could lead humanity out of the pandemic through its R&D prowess. Critical questions and concerns around who may gain financially from vaccine development, whether these gains would be justified, and what 'good' exactly the public would get in return for the subsidies governments had channeled into the pharma industry's R&D laboratories, were often rebuffed by pointing to the public's dependence on the pharmaceutical industry for the provision and manufacture of a safe Covid-19 vaccine.

To understand how we got to a point where the market seems to be the chief creator and curator of the public good in healthcare, let's take a step back. The Covid-19 pandemic has hit humankind at a point in time where many healthcare systems have been increasingly "marketized", as part of a broader historical move toward neoliberal governance regimes across public life

(Amable 2010). Differing in degrees to which it was embraced in different countries and taking place over decades, marketization happened through three interrelated dynamics: the gradual defunding of public services, which left healthcare systems with little spare capacity, the increasing privatization of broad elements of the healthcare system, and the adoption of market tools, measures, and logics in those domains that remained under public management (e.g. Zuiderent-Jerak 2009; Caduff 2020; Mason and Araujo 2020—see also Prainsack and Wagenaar in this volume, Chapter 9). In neoclassical economic thinking, markets allocate resources and property rights, balance out supply and demand, and establish a price where value for both parties is maximized. Such markets are said to be efficient and effective. In *these* markets, all the effects or "externalities" that the market creates are absorbed by its own pricing mechanisms, and a market's boundaries draw a relatively clear line between what is "inside" and what is "outside" (Mountford and Geiger 2021)—and by extension what is a private or a public good.[1] However, as Arrow (1963) so poignantly noted over a half-century ago, like many other markets, healthcare markets are often far removed from this neoclassical ideal. As amply demonstrated through the Covid-19 pandemic, demand for vaccinations, medicines, or hospital beds is rarely predictable; essential need leads to little or no price elasticity; know-how is unevenly distributed; and the patenting regime further distorts the market and often prevents market access for the most vulnerable in society (Geiger and Gross 2018). Market failure in healthcare, then, is not an aberration but an everyday reality. Some of these market failures may be worked out within the market itself. In spring 2020, manufacturers in the market for personal and protective equipment, for instance, quickly responded to shortages caused by the pandemic's global onset by increasing production, and new entrants repurposed manufacturing equipment for clothing or sports gear lying idle. In other areas, regulation and public governance may be able to alleviate the most obvious failures, safeguarding central aspects of the public good or at least preventing the worst "bads" (or negative externalities, in economists' speak). The European Union's (EU) pledge, in early summer 2020, to ensure "universal access to tests, treatments and vaccines against coronavirus and for the global recovery," represents one example of a "private" good being overlayed with (global) collective concerns.[2]

These few examples abundantly highlight that the healthcare market is never "just" a market but that its economy will always and forever be a *moral* and *political* economy. Thus, when personal and protective equipment started to be in short supply in March and April 2020, responding to these

4 MARKETIZATION AND THE COLLECTIVE GOOD

shortages became not just a logistical and manufacturing issue. It became a political target and show of national strength; it also became a social allocation conundrum, for instance in discussions around whether private nursing homes would be provided with personal and protective equipment by the state. And while negotiating with the major pharma manufacturers for advance purchase agreements of promising Covid-19 vaccines in confidential market arrangements, the EU and other world leaders also knew that shutting out the rest of the world from procuring these vaccines would ultimately be counter-productive (though this did not stop them from doing so). It is in the encounter and clashes between these different facets of healthcare—as a political entity, as a market object, and as a societal concern—that morality is being negotiated, struggles for the collective good take place, and civil society voices can be heard or suppressed. Thus, where Brown and Zavestoski (2004) locate an important motor for healthcare social movements in countering the "scientization" of medical decision making, this volume focally considers the market and its governance in fueling public discourses and in triggering certain types of healthcare activism (though, as I will explain below, scientific and economic dynamics are inseparable—a certain kind of science always presupposes a certain kind of economic governance).

2. Activists and Their Struggles for the Collective Good

The World Health Organization states that "the enjoyment of the highest attainable standard of health is one of the fundamental rights of every human being" (www.who.int). Yet, the attainment of this human right has been and still is an elusive goal for many. Activism typically arises from this rights-based conception of healthcare in those places where individuals or communities find this right violated, for instance where medicines or healthcare services are prohibitively expensive or not available at all. In many cases, activists emerge among those individuals or communities who are most directly impacted by having their rights to healthcare access inhibited—people with illnesses and their families (see Rabeharisoa and Doganova's Chapter 3 for a brief historical overview of patient activism). While patient advocacy in all its facets is a central aspect of healthcare activism, a broader take, adopted in this book, includes individuals or collectives concerned with healthcare issues even if not personally affected, as for instance parts of the Access to Medicines movement. Brown and Zavestoski (2004, 679) utilize the term "health social movements" in their classic paper on the topic, which they define as "collective challenges to medical policy, public health policy and politics, belief systems, research and practice which include an array of formal and informal organizations, supporters, networks of cooperation and media." They categorize these health social movements into "embodied" movements (focused on the personal experience of illness), "access" movements (seeking equitable access to healthcare), and "constituency-based" movements (for instance women's health or environmental justice movements). While broadly concurring with their definition, my preference for the word "activism" rather than "social movement" aims to signal the sometimes precarious state of the collectives that carry out the "activist" activities. Where "social movement" conjures up images of large and relatively well-organized networks potentially spread over many different organizations, the term activism fully recognizes the political dimension of such collective action yet also acknowledges that this action may not always be carried out by a highly organized or indeed internally cohesive grouping. The term "activism" also implies that change and contest can emanate from so-called "challenger" positions outside the market as well as from institutional insiders (Woodhouse et al. 2002; Martin 2007) – Geiger's (2017) example of 'physician activists' would be a case in point. These actions may remain local and fleeting, as for instance when citizens protest against the closure of a local hospital, but they always include what Martin (2007) calls "direct action": a clear critique and contestation of the institutional status quo.

We should note two points raised by Martin (2007, 24): first, not all those who engage in activism would use or even appreciate the label, with some considering their actions as "simply doing what is necessary to address a pressing problem." In fact, in the empirical research done as part of our ERC MISFIRES project (grant agreement no. 771217), the label "activist" is one that is often critically debated by our diverse research participants. And second, activism is always embedded in specific and situated "ecologies of activism," only able to blossom if a supporting, interested, or open context can be created.

So, what do healthcare activists aim to achieve? Specific goals can of course vary dramatically, and this book's chapters provide a small snapshot into this variety. Yet, I argue that by and large all of the healthcare activists presented in these pages have a guiding vision of what I will call the "collective good"—a vision of what is "moral" or "right." In this volume, these visions include advocating for improved testing technology, creating awareness about genetic predispositions to breast cancer, protesting egregious pharmaceutical pricing practices, and "hacking" proprietary medical devices. Much of the time, while representing a powerful driver, what "good" exactly it is that activists are

6 MARKETIZATION AND THE COLLECTIVE GOOD

aiming to defend remains implicit in the practices they engage in, and it may be left to the analyst to explicate it. In addition, a particular definition of the collective good may be unique to a particular grouping, and one that may or may not correspond to others' definitions – a vision of a particular "collective" good may thus not necessarily correspond to a "common" or a "public" one. Even in the same activist grouping there are likely to be fractional divisions as to the definition of the collective good and how to achieve this, as Stendahl and Geiger (2020) demonstrate through the example of a "flanked" diabetes 1 patient movement (see also Gottlieb in this volume, Chapter 8).

In some cases, the notion of the collective good is actively foregrounded, and in those cases it is frequently confounded with homonyms such as the common or public good. For instance, at the time of writing this introduction, in late 2020, the distribution and rollout of Covid-19 vaccinations were planned. Aware of the potential inequalities in access depending on where in the world one lived, healthcare activists called for any Covid-19 vaccine to become a "global public good," available and affordable to every last citizen of the planet. The phrase was soon adopted by public officials including United Nations Secretary-General Antonio Guterres and World Health Organization Director-General Dr Tedros Adhanom Ghebreyesus, though often what exactly was meant with it remained unclear.[3] A public good, according to Paul Samuelson's (1954) classic definition, is a good that is non-rivalrous (one person's consumption of the good does not subtract from another's) and non-excludable, meaning that a person cannot feasibly be prevented from access to the good. The public good, then, truly is the property of all; it is the most collective of all goods. Yet, as Samuelson himself readily admitted, "pure" public goods are in fact relatively rare cases—examples often mentioned are clean air, the light from a lighthouse, or national defense—and the difference between public and private goods may in fact be one of degree rather than binary opposition. From that perspective, vaccines, treatments, ventilator access, or hospital beds may be objects of public *costs* or expenditure. However, because they are at least partly rivalrous and excludable, and in fact often supplied through conventional market mechanisms, they could never be true public goods. By contrast, the herd immunity created through widespread vaccination rollouts would be a public good, as would a notion of healthcare and wellbeing for all (see Love 2020).

In fact, in many cases calls for the "public good" by activists or public figures are a shorthand to signal the need for more, or more targeted, public or civic involvement in biomedical markets—as in the orphan drug reimbursement cases that Rabeharisoa and Doganova (Chapter 3) and Moran and Mountford

(Chapter 4) consider. In these cases, activists advocate for different versions and visions of what I call the "collective good"—goods where individual and communal (or private and public) value and economic and moral reasoning are intrinsically intertwined. The term collective good, which I put forward in this volume, points to the entanglements and overlaps between "rights" and "goods" from a moral philosophical perspective (Hummel and Braun 2020). It also highlights that the way collective goods are construed depends on how the community advocating for it is defined (Widdows and Cordell 2011), and of course on the practices that a particular community engages in and the values it holds. Though we do not adopt her terminology, Elinor Ostrom's related term of a "common pool good" also reminds us that there is in fact a "commons" and thus a degree of collective ownership, control, or governance associated with a collective good (Ostrom and Ostrom 2015; Prainsack 2019).

As a working assumption for this volume, I thus postulate that the collective good in healthcare activism becomes shaped and defined in the activists' practices – specifically by the discursive and/or embodied negotiations over the collective value of biomedical products and services through which a collective seeks to gain a certain level of control over the economic ordering and governance of that good. This definition de-emphasizes the question of property rights, which is at the forefront of both economic and legal definitions of notions of the public or the common good. Instead, it highlights the more active and dynamic nature of a good that is always under negotiation, but where this negotiation at least partly relates to the economic organization of that good (including its innovation, valuation, and distribution). It also leaves space both for cases where this "good" is a material one that can have property rights attached (a "people's vaccine," for instance, where patent rights are held as a collective property), *and* more conceptual notions of what is "good" for a given collective, as for instance in the attempts to safeguard public innovation spaces in biomedical research.

3. Multiple Concerns—Multiple Goods?

A number of theoretical frameworks may help conceptualize the struggles for the collective good in and around healthcare markets. McLoughlin et al. (2017) and Sharon (2018) for instance utilize Boltanski and Thévenot's framework of orders of worth (1991/2006)[4] to illustrate how healthcare is answerable to arguments belonging to different justificatory regimes. Boltanski and Thévenot (2006) point toward the fact that individuals bring a shared

8 MARKETIZATION AND THE COLLECTIVE GOOD

sense of what is good or worthy to any public dispute, and they present six broad orders that social actors fall back on when constructing judgments and evaluations of other actors, objects, or a situation (the market; the industrial; the domestic; the civic; the inspired; and fame). While these six orders are coherent spheres of evaluation in and of themselves, Boltanski and Thévenot emphasize that they can and often do co-exist in the same social context. In fact, they may be selectively and pragmatically mobilized by actors to justify or contest certain valuations or judgments (Boltanski and Thévenot 2000). These orders can thus be deployed flexibly to cope with tensions and conflicts in evolving situations. Most of the time, compromises can be found between orders, but there may also be situations where these orders are irreconcilable and a common moral ground may not be established. McLoughlin et al. (2017) for instance detect clashes in healthcare between four orders of worth: the domestic (care for the sick), the civic (citizens' rights and voice), the industrial (healthcare as an efficient socio-technical system), and the market (patients-as-consumers; price as the ultimate arbiter). Sharon (2018) identifies a similar conflict when large multinational technology firms such as Google or Apple move into health research. Rather than pitching an "amoral" market worth against a (more) moral civic register, she argues that different conceptions of the collective good are negotiated through several justificationary regimes, each with their own articulation of what is moral (in her case the market, the civic, the industrial, the project, and a "vitalist" one).

While we do not follow Boltanski and Thévenot's orders of worth framework explicitly in this volume, we take from their analyses the need to understand the "market" element of healthcare not necessarily in opposition to but in continuous interaction and exchange with other ways of seeing and judging what is moral or "good" for a given collective. Thus, rather than drawing any simple dichotomies between "markets" and "morals," these moralities and ways of conceptualizing the collective good are often overlayed. For instance, many EU healthcare policies are arguably driven by the belief that market competition is a central force for innovation and over the longer term lead to societal benefits, yet they also acknowledge the need to steer the market's creation of the collective good through public engagement and regulation (Geiger 2020).

Emphasizing how markets can in fact benefit through taking account of diverse conceptions of the collective good, my colleagues and I have previously argued that healthcare could be conceived as a "concerned" market–markets where multiple actors' values and concerns clash (Geiger et al. 2014). Such markets can never be represented through a single perspective of "what is good." Nor indeed is there one view of when such a market's workings need to change in the interest of the collective good, or one way to change them. Rather, these markets are deeply contested by a great diversity of actors with equally diverse perspectives and value measures, all grappling to frame and engage in economic and non-economic exchanges where multiple value registers meet. These clashes of values and morals force a level of reflexivity onto the market and open up the possibility that these clashes can be publicly articulated and negotiated. Callon et al. (2009) have proposed the use of hybrid forums as reflective spaces of physical or virtual encounter in which heterogeneous actors—concerned publics, experts, politicians—collectively define the problems in which they are all implicated and search for solutions. Other forms of deliberative democracy have also been invoked in healthcare (Davies et al. 2006; see also Prainsack and Wagenaar in this volume). The question of how to build these hybrid forums to voice multiple conceptions and definitions of the collective good is a recurring theme in several of the book's chapters, for instance in Galasso and Geiger's conceptual piece on patient and public involvement (Chapter 2), but also in Lindén's description of cervical cancer activists (Chapter 6) and in Rabeharisoa and Doganova's tracing of orphan disease patients' pricing battles through evidence-based activism (Chapter 3).

4. Hearing Multiple Voices

There can be immediate pragmatic effects of opening up the negotiation of the collective good in healthcare markets to multiple voices. As mentioned above, during the Covid-19 pandemic an often maligned pharmaceutical industry has arguably received a considerable image boost by being heralded by some as our only potential savior to free society from a lengthy period of personal restrictions and economic hardship (e.g. Lowry 2020). For many, tinkering with the way the pharmaceutical market is structured became almost unthinkable, as became obvious during the lengthy negotiations at the World Trade Organization over a patent waiver for Covid-19 vaccines. At the same time, the pandemic did provide an opportunity to question and reflect on some of the industry's "sacred cows" (Scholz and Smith 2020): private governance of R&D processes even when these are partly publicly funded, intellectual property protection, and profit-maximizing pricing strategies. Though these practices had been standard industry practice for decades and criticized myriad times before the pandemic, they were now openly debated as jeopardizing the

10 MARKETIZATION AND THE COLLECTIVE GOOD

collective good, defined as broad and affordable access to coronavirus medications and/or vaccines, rapid innovation, and open sharing of scientific insights. Just as the pharmaceutical industry was elevated from a position of commercial supplier to the public health sector to a central societal actor, the crisis also foregrounded some of its typically invisible market practices and made them subject to public debate—as practices that must contribute not just to shareholders' bottom line but also (and perhaps predominantly) to the collective good. Opening up these debates had immediate consequences in some cases. For instance, following controversies over the price point at which the Covid-19 treatment candidate remdesivir would be made available in different countries, the pharmaceutical maker Gilead's chief executive officer Daniel O'Day felt compelled to publish an open letter responding to criticism that Gilead may be profiteering from its invention at the expense of global health concerns.[5] The letter stated that the company was fully aware of its responsibilities "to ensure price is in no way a hindrance to ensuring rapid and broad treatment," and that it would price remdesivir below what it would normally charge for a treatment of its kind.[6]

Beyond these (relatively rare) immediate effects, providing space for multiple conceptions of the collective good in healthcare is also vital in the long run. As Moran and Mountford argue in Chapter 4 of this volume, marketization is a process where the market's logics, values, institutions, and culture obliterate or at least weaken alternative conceptions of public life and social exchange.[7] Brown (2015, 31) explains this with reference to Michel Foucault's work: "neoliberal rationality disseminates the model of the market to all domains and activities—even where money is not at issue—and configures human beings exhaustively as market actors, always, only, and everywhere as homo economicus." Marketization, in this sense, can lead to a point where the market logic is used implicitly or explicitly to value and evaluate persons, situations, events, choices, or encounters in such terms as return on investment, efficiency, competition, or human capital, to the detriment of other alternative moralities or values. Thus, even a fully public healthcare system can be heavily marketized in its logics and its practices, and individuals contribute to this marketization by becoming "invested" in this rationality. Activists do not—and perhaps cannot—automatically stand outside this market logic, but importantly they attempt to insert their conceptions of the collective good into the market's governance structures. Indeed, Rabeharisoa and Doganova argue that their rare disease patient groups are deeply involved with the pharmaceutical market—not as dupes or hostages, but as active participants and shaping forces, bringing vital evidence and knowledge into the market. Of course, this also means that these activists may in fact walk a moral tightrope. On the one hand, by engaging with "the market" and its moralities, there is a constant risk of cooptation: that becoming conversant with the logic of the market and engaging in dialogue to stem its excesses or rectify its overflows means adopting its rationality, thus cementing the market as a preeminent institution responsible for providing the collective good. In the extreme, this includes the risk of biomedical companies doing just enough 'good' in order to "neutralize dissent" (Ismail and Kamat 2018, 569). One example of such neutralization of patient dissent are Compassionate Use patient programs, where a proportion of a drug manufacturer's medicines is allocated free of charge or at very low cost to patients in need, which may silence broader, systemic calls for a reform of the pharmaceutical pricing model in the face of often egregious medication prices.[8] On the other hand, attempting to find compromises between the logic of the market and those emanating from different perspectives may often be the only route to achieve change in a world where alternatives to the neoliberal order have become almost unthinkable.

5. Marketized *and* Personalized—Medical Science and the Collective Good

Up to this point we have ignored a central issue in our argument: that healthcare's morals and markets are always intrinsically linked to the evolution of scientific and clinical practice. Dynamics and shifts in these practices may both influence conceptions of the collective good and the economic orders through which biomedical innovations reach patients (Clarke et al. 2003). Though often seen as different spheres, the scientific and the economic orders are thus better conceived as non-identical twins, as they typically emanate from the same (ideological) stock. Jasanoff and colleagues famously proposed in 2004 that "the ways in which we know and represent the world ... are inseparable from the way in which we choose to live in it." In short, science, society, and its markets are co-produced: the types of technologies and techniques that dominate a scientific domain at any one moment also presuppose and/or cement certain economic and social orderings.

Two scientific shifts have in recent times most heavily influenced conceptions of the collective good in healthcare and simultaneously created widespread changes in biomedical markets: the move toward precision or "personalized" medicine through advances in molecular and genomic medicine, and, relatedly, a broader "datafication" of individuals' health and other personal traces (Hoeyer et al. 2019). Often subsumed under the label of data-driven medicine, both of these techno-scientific developments have become pet targets of public and economic policy over the past ten years. President Barack Obama famously heralded the dawn of a new healthcare age characterized by both processes when launching one of the leading initiatives on precision medicine, "All of Us," which would assist in tailoring healthcare "to individuals' lifestyles, genes, environment and preferences" (White House 2015). While undoubtedly promising important innovations, these scientific developments have been heavily shaped by private companies, including some of the largest and most powerful corporate entities in the world ('Big Tech' and 'Big Pharma'), who have quickly outpaced all but a handful of large public institutions in their push toward precision medicine. This is an almost necessary economic consequence of a simple scientific fact: data-driven medicine relies on an unprecedented scale of data access, collection, storage, and analysis at a time where the digital and pharmaceutical domains have witnessed unprecedented corporate concentration of power (Hogle 2016). Thus, if the future collective good in healthcare is cast in terms of data-driven medicine, then it is almost inevitable that this good will be channeled through market orders dominated by large, private organizations.

Critics of neoliberalism see this future scale- and data-driven biomedical marketplace as reducing the patient, and often the healthcare provider, to "knowledge-producing machines" or "subroutines" (Nik-Khah 2018). These would feed a marketplace where knowledge is generated and accumulated "not to create more knowledge available for all, but instead the right kind of knowledge selected for its usefulness to (because demanded by) well-heeled patrons" (2018, 94). Thus, many critical voices argue that the personalization and datafication of biomedicine leads to an increase in *private* goods rather than *collective* ones, even if it is individuals' and collectives' data that feed this particular medical economy (Hummel and Braun 2020; Geiger and Gross 2021). This may even be the case when private corporations cooperate with public bodies in so-called public–private partnership arrangements, such as public–private genomics initiatives where the private entity gains property rights over large and publicly sourced accumulations of individuals' DNA data (Galasso and Geiger 2021). Of course, such partnerships are purportedly always forged in the service of keeping the precarious balance between economic and collective concerns. Yet, in many cases, it remains unclear whether the potential future value to the public truly balances out the costs of the partnerships in terms of governments handing decision-making power and property rights to private entities (Powles and Hodson 2017). At the very least, in charging private entities with public innovation goals, governments risk further consolidating the hegemony of the market's morals—and with it, arguably cementing the belief that only the market can deliver the collective good. To put it simply, the more sophisticated and "bigger" medical science becomes, the more challenging it will be to argue against the fact that the private market is the only thinkable place where the collective good can be shaped.

6. Defending the Collective Good in the Age of "Me" Medicine

The increasing power and influence of private "big data" or "big science" entities on innovation trajectories and decision making in healthcare is an important factor in explaining some of the current activist struggles described within this volume, and it is one that Prainsack and Wagenaar critically discuss in their concluding Chapter 9. Yet, the move to ever more costly and data-intensive medical sciences also has subtler consequences on the assembling of collective voices in healthcare. In discussing precision medicine and genomic sciences, Dickenson (2013) famously diagnosed the move from a "we" medicine to a "me" medicine. Dickenson sees neoliberalism's traces in personalized biomedical approaches acting to push individualist thinking in healthcare and weaken communitarian views, especially in the persistent rhetoric affirming individual choice in healthcare as an absolute value. While autonomy and a right to decision making in healthcare contexts are generally recognized as essential, pushing this autonomy rhetorically into the notion of choice, as often framed by the biomedical industry, turns it into de facto consumerism: where healthcare products and organizational structures become increasingly marketized or market-like, Dickenson argues, the patient assumes the default position of individual consumer. Even if one does not buy into a "consumerist" interpretation of current healthcare models, the ever narrower stratification of disease categories and associated illness groups makes the assembly of truly collective voices a difficult undertaking—the more "personalized" healthcare gets, the more fragmented the collectively concerned voices may become (though see Prainsack 2018).

The often lauded "unprecedented" ability for data analysis and ever more minute stratification of patient and illness categories does not only distract from a communal view of healthcare to the advantage of an individualistic one. This ability also turns the responsibility for (ill) health away from fate or bad luck toward putting patients "in charge" of their own destiny as (neoliberal) entrepreneurs of the self, as Cheded and Hopkinson powerfully illustrate in their Chapter 7. Rather than encouraging a solidaristic or even activist perspective of tackling the root causes of many diseases, which may at least partly lie in socio-economic factors rather than individual ones, this prevention paradigm leads more typically to the responsibilization of individuals as "proto" patients who assiduously track individual risks and acceptable behaviors. Needless to say, in *this* healthcare universe, there is little space nor really any need for collective action—the market endogenizes all possible points of friction in the rhetorical trajectory from patient empowerment to fully individualized consumer choice (Mold 2015). Or, as Brown (2015, 38) puts it, "the subject is at once in charge of itself, responsible for itself, yet an instrumentalizable and potentially dispensable element of the whole. In this regard, the liberal democratic social contract is turning inside out." In this future scenario, the collective good is, at best, an aggregate of individual entitlements rather than a communitarian goal that would drive collective action. Regarding recent events, it remains to be seen whether Covid-19 and the associated government actions will trigger a (re)turn to collective responsibility and an awareness that true "collective goods" require collective involvement and governance.

Of course, the tension between individual freedom and collective good is nothing new. Neither is the fact that the collective good is always precarious, often disputed, and prone to capture by commercial interests (Boyle 2003). The boundaries between the invisible hand of the market, as governor of private goods, and the more visible one of the public actor, who represents society as shepherd of the collective good and shaper of the private one, have long been shown to be porous. And, as argued previously, many healthcare activists have in fact been engaging with and embedding their own conceptions of the collective good into the fabric of the biomedical industry. Market actors, meanwhile, have started counting on these patient groups for their "ethical citizenship" (Rose and Novas 2005). As mentioned before, what used to be seen as "hostile worlds"—those of private firms and those of civil society and activists, so acutely opposed for instance in the early days of AIDS activism (Epstein 1996)—have arguably become more and more entangled with the biomedicalization of healthcare (Clarke et al. 2003; Rabeharisoa 2003). And where this entanglement is missing, organizations often actively strive to create or regain it, as in Galasso and Geiger's discussion of patient and public involvement practices in genomics initiatives in Chapter 2. Where activists' conceptions of the collective good become enmeshed in the economic functioning of the market, activists are no longer "problematic" for that market—they are in fact needed to bolster the market's moral fabric. The problematic parties are the ones who refuse to make themselves calculable in this entangled "concerned market" frame. In current times, the most visible, vocal, and controversial of such "problematic" persons are the anti-vaccination activists and Covid skeptics who protest against what they see as big business/big government "dictating" individual responsibility for the greater good. In a sense, these particular "activists" have taken individualization to its ultimate degree and turned it against what they see as a state/market cabal that forces a notion of collective good onto them.

We can thus draw an idealized continuum from "invited activism," which directly serves to inject a certain level of moral legitimacy into market-based institutions, to "tolerated activism" by health activists who recognize the market and work to make it more moral by innovating, improving, or taming it, all the way to "deviant activists" who refuse to reconcile their moral worlds with those of the market and prefer to keep them "hostile." Again, this is not to say that all activists or patient representatives working within market-based institutions are either "pro"-market, captured, or unaware of the tightrope they are balancing. Most are very aware of the difficulties of working within a market-based system but choose to do so consciously to achieve their collective good objectives. This broad and idealized categorization also does not mean that "tolerated" activism cannot still take the form of "spectacular political protest and opposition" (Wehling et al. 2014, 240). We see such opposition in Moran and Mountford's Chapter 4 in the case of parents demonstrating in front of the Irish parliament for reimbursement of their children's specialty medicines; even if these demonstrations came to benefit the pharmaceutical industry that charged "economically inefficient" prices in the first place. But it is to say that healthcare activism is perhaps at its most provoking when it rejects a market-driven formulation of the collective good altogether.[9]

Let me summarize this introduction's argument before moving on to present the book's individual contributions: We live in an era where the collective good in healthcare is defined through diverse concerns but often channeled through "the market"—both as an institution and as an overarching logic of economic ordering and governance. As we move further and further into the realm of data-driven or precision medicine, this market logic is likely to occupy an increasingly central role in providing, steering, and governing the collective good in healthcare on behalf of the community. As this happens,

16   MARKETIZATION AND THE COLLECTIVE GOOD

space for negotiating and debating a truly collective good through multiple voices may shrink, but the entanglement of activist voice and market through "invited" or "tolerated" activism may also act to keep collective good concerns alive in an increasingly privatized and individualized market realm. And, as Prainsack and Wagenaar in their Chapter 9 so powerfully argue, with the devastations wrought by the Covid-19 pandemic there comes the hope that civil society and governments will in fact emerge with a common realization of just how necessary it is to defend and uphold spaces for a multivocal negotiation of the collective good in healthcare.

The contributors in this book volume and I are far from naively claiming that "all" healthcare activism is inherently good or justified, or that activists' definitions of the collective good are always morally superior (or indeed much different) from that of other stakeholders. Yet, acknowledging multiple concerns, even if some of these may be contested (as in the current case of Covid-19 vaccination skeptics) serves an important societal and moral function. In their "archeological" work of deconstructing naturalized processes, science and technology studies scholars often pose counterfactual questions. What would society look like if certain publics weren't around; what would happen, and who (if anyone) would fill the gap? Let's adopt this thought experiment: if "invited" activists, who are for instance involved in specific organizations' patient engagement initiatives, did not exist, these organizations would be devoid of valuable learning opportunities, and the activists themselves would be without designated forums to help govern the good produced by these organizations. If "tolerated" activists such as patient groups fighting for access to medicines or inclusion in clinical trials were to disappear, the market as a whole and its governance would risk becoming unmoored from collective good considerations that are outside their immediate sight. Though perhaps the least "heard" or acknowledged, "deviant" activists also fulfill an important purpose, in continually reminding us that the current economic organization of healthcare is but one of many possible ways of governing the collective good, and that "other worlds" are in fact conceivable (Roelvink 2015).

7. This Book's Contributions

While not all of the following chapters touch on all of the issues raised above, together they present a vivid array of civil society, patient groups, and other voices struggling to define and defend the collective good in the era of marketized, personalized, and datafied healthcare. In positioning themselves in relation to these dynamics, the activist and advocate groups we will encounter over the course of the next eight chapters at times adopt the vocabulary and tools proffered by the market, but in doing so inevitably contribute to shaping its meaning and form. As Moran and Mountford (Chapter 4) show us, for instance, engaging directly with market concerns such as pricing both expands the activists' remit and puts them at risk of being captured by "the market"; claiming a position of "empowerment," vis-à-vis regulators and commercial actors, as the T1D hackers in Gottlieb's account (Chapter 8), also runs the danger of being "uber compliant" to a neoliberal discourse. Thus, in the round, the individual chapters demonstrate that activists cannot ever fully escape the market in healthcare and its broader economic and institutional dynamics—but also highlight the significant role they play by defining and defending their own conceptions of the collective good vis-à-vis market-based organizations.

Several of the chapters in this volume engage with the notion of invited activism, pinpointing the opportunities but also potential difficulties patient groups face in being "welcomed" into the market's structure. Leading into this issue conceptually in Chapter 2, Ilaria Galasso and Susi Geiger present a contribution that acts as a counterintuitive to those chapters that focus more on "uninvited" activism. Utilizing Hirschmann's classic distinction between voice, exit, and loyalty, they argue that in most cases healthcare represents a classic "no exit" situation: while (limited) choice may exist as to providers or specific products and services, the decision *not* to engage at all with the healthcare market typically doesn't arise. On the contrary, much healthcare activism, as described by other chapters in this volume and epitomized by the HIV/AIDS movement in the 1980s, can be characterized as health *access* movements, to use Brown and Zavestoski's (2004) distinction. These movements typically fight for their constituents to gain entry into healthcare markets or to create a market around their illness in the first place, often working with policy makers, researchers, and pharmaceutical firms to make these markets happen. Of course, health access movements are not automatically pro-market advocates, to the contrary. The PXE community briefly described by Rabeharisoa and Doganova in their chapter for instance was careful to implement market governance mechanisms that would allow sharing of the intellectual property created in their collaborations with scientists and drugs firms, thus introducing an important collective good concern into market-based R&D processes.

The dynamics around access in precision medicine initiatives are different. Precision medicine initiatives are reliant on patient and public volunteering of the "raw materials" for the development of future biomedical markets. As

18 MARKETIZATION AND THE COLLECTIVE GOOD

Galasso and Geiger point out, for individuals who are unable to expect immediate returns from precision medicine initiatives in the form of immediately available products or services , the "costs" of contributing to these initiatives by donating their data or genetic samples often outweigh potential gains. As a consequence, "exit" or opt-out—refusing to participate—is by far easier than exercising voice to shape these initiatives for collective good concerns, which is almost absent from these initiatives. To avoid becoming more and more removed from the concerns of their stakeholders, many of these initiatives thus recreate voice and "invite" activism in the shape of patient and public involvement. Importantly, the lengths some of these organizations go through to institute these initiatives indirectly highlight the vital role that patient and public voices play in keeping biomedical markets and market practices imbued with collective good concerns.

Where Galasso and Geiger ask why certain healthcare organizations actively seek to engage with activist patients, Vololona Rabeharisoa and Liliana Doganova, in their Chapter 3, pose the reverse question: Why and how do patient organizations engage with the biomedical market? The authors locate the current struggles around intellectual property rights and prices of medicines in the context of an evolving "war on disease." "War on disease" highlights the epistemic role that patient organizations have adopted since the 1980s, which has in recent years extended into (co-) producing "market" knowledge—specifically knowledge around the value, costs, and pricing of economic entities. Through evidence-based activism, patient organizations, in the authors' account, are active actors within the markets they have helped create: "these patient organizations do not reject the market as a way to access drugs. Quite the contrary: For them, caring about the market is part and parcel of caring about the patients." Rabeharisoa and Doganova paint a brief historical arc of the development of patient movements from the advent of "experiential" knowledge in the 1940s and 1950s, through pursuing identity objectives in the 1960s, to a foregrounding of patient organizations' epistemic role in the 1980s to what Rabeharisoa et al. (2014) have coined "evidence-based activism." "War on disease" at this point shifted the very contours of which knowledge is seen as relevant and legitimate in the first place—and this soon included market knowledge. Thus, the rare disease patient organizations engage with economic entities such as cost, price, or value for money not as a reaction against market forces, but as a series of situated responses to difficulties in accessing medicines and establishing a "fair price" in a market that they have actively contributed to create.

The issue of a "fair price" and the clash of market and civic logics to arrive at such an elusive entity also stands at the center of Gillian Moran and Nicola Mountford's Chapter 4, who continue the context of rare disease patient groups encountered in Chapter 3. The authors zoom in on two specific social media campaigns, set in the aftermath of negative reimbursement decisions by the Irish health technology assessment unit (the National Centre for Pharmacoeconomics). Their chapter elucidates the mechanisms through which patient communities oppose and eventually manage to reverse government decisions for the orphan drugs Orkambi and Spinraza. While social media are often accused of creating a "shout loudest" culture, Moran and Mountford demonstrate that through careful enrolment of other—previously "unconcerned"—actors and media, the campaigns systematically promulgate a valuation logic that stands apart from the economic valuations cemented by extant market governance practices. A tension arises from their chapter, of particular relevance to the volume's overall concern: on the one hand, by forcing the government's hand to reimburse highly expensive medications, the activities of the two patient communities arguably played directly into the hands of the pharmaceutical industry. The quick succession of both cases, only a year apart, further begs the question of whether these "spectacular" protestations can have any longer-term impact on the system itself. At the same time, campaigns such as #YesOrkambi and #SpinrazaNow are vital to reiterate the broader concerns of actors who uphold a civic logic in the face of marketized economic evaluation processes—hopefully to the ultimate benefit of all those patient voices who may be less visible or audible but suffer no less from a purely market-driven conception of the collective good.

In Chapter 5, Klaus Hoeyer and Henriette Langstrup lead us into a consideration of what it means for the collective good to be continuously negotiated by introducing us to a healthcare system that has become "datafied." Hoeyer and Langstrup present us with a case where public activism is relatively muted. This is unsurprising, perhaps, as the case they are considering—the digitalization of Danish healthcare infrastructures—is strongly characterized by collaborative governance mechanisms and full of the "invited" spaces that Galasso and Geiger reflect on in their chapter. In fact, the Danish government goes to great lengths to make *sundhed.dk*, the online portal giving access to the public health data infrastructure, as useful and "empowering" to individuals as possible. Yet, dissenting voices do come to the fore in moments of breakdown or "ruination," as the authors put it. They show that "failure" does not just happen in markets but in processes of public organizing too; however, they also demonstrate that these moments of breakdown open up a cycle that can lead from ruination to repair (and to further promise). Hoeyer and Langstrup discuss the moral ambiguity of state-sanctioned empowerment where patients and other stakeholders who are engaged in various forms of activism attempt to affect public digital data infrastructures. They also show how activists-turned-collaborators in the datafication project became "agents of repair" in their own right. Their focus on the never-ending work of "infrastructuring" also emphasizes the epistemological ambiguity of these attempts to affect and govern data flows as collective goods: what exactly this collective good is and how it can be arrived at is always and forever a contested issue.

Lisa Lindén continues the focus on "epistemic politics" through participation in healthcare governance in Chapter 6—though in contrast to Hoeyer and Langstrup's mostly "invited" Danish activists, Lindén's Swedish gynecological cancer activists (the "GCG") have to fight for a seat at the table. Similar to Rabeharisoa and Doganova's rare disease patients, they gain this seat through evidence-based activism—even if, as Lindén shows, this knowledge can still be highly contested. This evidence is then used by the activists to occupy a broad set of patient advocacy roles, including those of "initiators," "controllers," and "influencers." Thus, the policy change process is "policed" by the advocates at every step, but these roles, explains Lindén, can only be understood in dynamic relation to other actors, including policy makers and (presumably, though not explicitly mentioned) biomedical industry. Her account shows how defining the collective good is indeed a collective and embodied achievement "enacted in and through practices, rather than being an abstract construction based on general ethical or political principles." The activities of patient groups, in this reading, can thus never be divorced from the dynamics in the larger socio-material assemblages in which they take place.

This point is also brought into stark relief by Mohammed Cheded and Gillian Hopkinson's Chapter 7 on breast cancer patients' roles and the dynamics of individualization and collectivism that different narratives of these roles create. Cheded and Hopkinson describe two alternative breast cancer social movement narratives across the three illness phases of pre-cancer, illness, and post-illness. The mainstream narrative formats a role of the responsibilized, heteronormative biosocial citizen whose fate is intrinsically linked to accepting, adhering to, and promoting the biomedical explanation of their illness. As becomes apparent throughout Cheded and Hopkinson's account, in the shadows of this narrative lurks a significant level of governmentality of the individual patient, partly driven by market forces that keep a shadowy existence in the funding drives, the pink ribbon campaigns, and the consumerist tools that help survivors restore their former selves in line with this narrative.

As the authors mention, breast cancer is the top pharmaceutical investment therapeutic category—though it is not the biggest global killer—and is typically seen as a highly "lucrative" disease area by the industry itself.[10] It is telling that the biomedical (and other) markets are at once nowhere and everywhere in this narrative—where a faulty gene is the narrative's "villain," the "heroes" are those industries that work to detect, predict, and fight this villain. As Cheded and Hopkinson point out, the alternative to this mainstream narrative, proffered by "deviant" activists in the vocabulary used above, proposes a much more critical, non-normative, and non-market-compliant reading of the collective good in breast cancer activism. This narrative includes marginalized voices, those who have fallen victim to environmental harms caused by polluting industries, and those who are unable or unwilling to fit the molds offered by mainstream biomedical discourse. Cheded and Hopkinson's account powerfully demonstrates how efforts to generalize an illness experience into commercially driven activist roles end up individualizing patients and in particular alienating those who do not recognize themselves in these narratives—those who don't feel "pink" enough, perhaps.

The penultimate Chapter 8, by Samantha Gottlieb, returns to this neoliberal shaping of the notion of patient empowerment and the challenges that activists face when reclaiming this notion. Gottlieb charts the balancing acts that type 1 diabetes "hackers" perform by working at the very boundaries of the medical device market and regulation when creating unregulated or "hacked" closed-loop insulin pumps and meters. Interestingly, Gottlieb notes that the very hackers who are spearheading a movement that could be emblematic for patient collectives reclaiming their agency from large biomedical firms in fact often have close ties to the medical device industry. Being at once inside and outside the market, for these advocates, is not mutually exclusive. Neither is being simultaneously uber-compliant (by taking on the neoliberal mantle of self-management) and non-compliant (by performing their own non-market version of being an empowered patient).

Gottlieb closes her contribution with an important reflection, which in many ways permeates other chapters too: though mostly born from desperation and necessity, patient activism that addresses market misfires all too often remains the purview of health-, economically, and digitally literate individuals—at least, this is the kind of activism that has been traced in the pages of this volume. I suggest that one explanation for this fact is an error of omission: that we as researchers tend to gravitate to those voices we most readily hear and see in public discourse; or indeed those in which we may recognize ourselves most closely. While this volume undoubtedly holds important insights into current dynamics of *this* type of healthcare activism, we should not forget that there are many more marginalized, unheard, or actively silenced patient and activist collectives, most of whom will forever remain "uninvited" by dominant institutions. It should be our future task as researchers to make those marginal voices stronger and provide a space for *their* conceptions of the collective good to be seen and heard. In an era where, for better or worse, biomedical markets need to concern everyone who comes in touch with healthcare, we should ensure that these markets also show concern for everyone, regardless of how far their individual and collective voices carry.

This call for an encompassing form of solidarity in healthcare and a renewed role for both state and civil society—and, I would add, activist researchers—in a post-Covid-19 world is made loud and clear by Barbara Prainsack and Hendrik Wagenaar in their concluding Chapter 9. Reflecting on recent and potential future changes caused by the Covid-19 pandemic on societies' "moral landscapes," the authors argue that the time has come to rethink the role of "the state" and its relation to civil society, within and beyond the context of the Covid-19 crisis. Prainsack and Wagenaar thus complete the arc drawn in this volume; an arc reaching from this introductory chapter's warning about the hegemony of a market logic in contemporary healthcare across the numerous entanglements between state, market, and civil society that the subsequent chapters demonstrate, to their own diagnosis that the ideology of public choice economics has failed the most vulnerable in this pandemic crisis. But there are ways to remediate this state of affairs. As they point out, many states have shown a level of innovativeness and assertiveness during the pandemic that have arguably been missing from preceding decades' deference to the market as chief healthcare innovator. Thus, where authors such as Mariana Mazzucato see a renewed role for the state as entrepreneur, Prainsack and Wagenaar call for it to reassert its role as *social* innovator. Yet, they are also clear in stating that this cannot be done without the collaboration of grassroots civil society. Thus, their chapter offers a hopeful ending to this book volume: beyond the devastation it has caused, maybe the current pandemic has opened up a window to rethink the collective good in healthcare beyond any facile juxtaposition of markets and morals.

I hope that this volume will demonstrate to its readers just how powerful a shaper and defender of the collective good healthcare activism is. Again, this is not a naïve stance to say that *all* healthcare activism is necessarily or intrinsically good. But by *concerning* themselves with and *caring about* the way healthcare is organized, activism opens up current biomedical structures, logics, and institutions for debate. By *caring about*, pushing for, and driving innovation in the market and the state, healthcare activists—be they patients, concerned publics, or experts—are an indispensable part of our fabric of the economic ordering of modern healthcare. Caring, in Puig de la Bellacasa's (2017, 12) sense, is always a speculative and political undertaking; it is fundamentally disruptive, seeking that which can be "as good as possible" by opening up "reconfigurations engaged with troubled presences." And even though, just like the healthcare activists we observe in this volume, as researchers we may sometimes play into and help consolidate existing economic power structures, caring about healthcare and the shape it takes is what this book volume is all about. Let it stir up a "troubled presence" in the moral and economic analysis of contemporary healthcare.

Acknowledgments

Susi Geiger has received funding for writing this chapter from the European Research Council (ERC) under the European Union's Horizon 2020 research and innovation programme (grant agreement No. 771217).

Notes

1. See Carrier and Miller (1998) or Callon (1998) for extended critiques of this "abstraction" and the role that such economic thought has played in shaping really existing markets.
2. https://global-response.europa.eu/index_en.
3. WHO Coronavirus Briefing 12 June 2020.
4. Boltanski and Thévenot (2006) point toward the fact that individuals bring a sense of what is good or worthy to any dispute, and they present six broad orders that social actors fall back on when constructing judgments and evaluations of other actors, objects, or a situation. These include: the market (where objects are evaluated from the angle of profit maximization and competition); the industrial (emphasizing science, productivity, and instrumental relationships); the domestic (which considers attachment, hierarchy, and honesty); the civic (valuing civic solidarity, the collective, and delegation); the inspired (emphasizing charisma, creation, and uniqueness); and an order of worth based on fame (reputation, public opinion, and success). While these six orders are coherent spheres of evaluation in and of themselves, Boltanski and Thévenot emphasize that they can and often do co-exist in the same social context. In fact, they may be selectively and pragmatically mobilized by actors to justify or contest certain valuations or judgments in different situations. Orders can thus be deployed to cope with tensions and conflicts in dynamic situations.
5. E.g. https://www.channelnewsasia.com/news/world/covid-19-coronavirus-gilead-price-drug-public-good-profit-12,709,990.

24　MARKETIZATION AND THE COLLECTIVE GOOD

6. https://stories.gilead.com/articles/an-open-letter-from-daniel-oday-june-29. The letter also emphasized that the relatively unusual pricing decision taken—to set a standard per patient price for developed countries—balanced out public good consideration with a long-term "public good" of continuing investment in R&D.
7. For a narrower definition of marketization see for instance Birch and Siemiatycki (2016).
8. On a sidenote, the fact that the allocation of these medicine programs is often done through a lottery system is often considered less than moral by the patients involved.
9. We may note in passing that such "alternative economies" are not as far-fetched or without precedent as one may think. In France, for instance, a large part of the pharmaceutical industry was under public ownership until the early 1990s (Bourgeron and Geiger 2020).
10. Phamaprojects Research Report, "Pharma R&D Annual Review 2019," https://pharmaintelligence.informa.com/~/media/informa-shop-window/pharma/2019/files/whitepapers/pharma-rd-review-2019-whitepaper.pdf, and QY Research Report 2020, "Global Breast Cancer Treatment Drugs Market," https://startupng.com.ng/uncategorized/123440/global-breast-cancer-treatment-drugs-marketlucrative-regions-for-the-manufacturers-in-2020-abbvie-abbott-bristol-myers-squibb/.

References

Amable, B. (2010), Morals and Politics in the Ideology of Neo-liberalism, *Socio-Economic Review*, 9:1, 3–30. doi:10.1093/ser/mwq015.

Arrow, K. J. (1963), Uncertainty and the Welfare Economics of Medical Care. *American Economic Review*, 53:5, 851–83.

Birch, K., and Siemiatycki, M. (2016), Neoliberalism and the Geographies of Marketization: The Entangling of State and Markets, *Progress in Human Geography*, 40:2, 177–98.

Boltanski, L., and Thévenot, L. (2000), The Reality of Moral Expectations: A Sociology of Situated Judgement, *Philosophical Explorations*, 3:3, 208–31.

Boltanski, L., and Thévenot, L. (2006), *On Justification: Economies of Worth*, Princeton University Press.

Bourgeron, T., and Geiger, S. (2020), Building Opacity, Fighting Opacity: The Opacification of Drug Prices in the EU's Pharmaceutical Market from the 1980s to 2019, 32nd Annual SASE Meeting.

Boyle, J. (2003), The Second Enclosure Movement and the Construction of the Public Domain, *Law and Contemporary Problems*, 66:1/2, 33–74.

Brown, P., and Zavestoski, S. (2004), Social Movements in Health: An Introduction, *Sociology of Health and Illness*, 26:6, 679–94.

Brown, W. (2015), *Undoing the Demos: Neoliberalism's Stealth Revolution*, Zone Books.

Caduff, C. (2020), What Went Wrong: Corona and the World after the Full Stop, *Medical Anthropology Quarterly*, 34:4, 467–87.

Callon, M. (ed.) (1998), *The Laws of the Markets*, Wiley-Blackwell.

Callon, M., Lascoumes, P., and Barthe, Y. (2009), *Acting in an Uncertain World: An Essay on Technical Democracy*, MIT Press.

Carrier, J. G., and Miller, D. (eds) (1998), *Virtualism: A New Political Economy*, Berg Publishers.

Clarke, A. E., Shim, J. K., Mamo, L., Fosket, J. R., and Fishman, J. R. (2003). Biomedicalization: Technoscientific Transformations of Health, Illness, and U.S. Biomedicine. *American Sociological Review*, 68:2, 161–94.

Davies, C., Wetherell, M., and Barnett, E. (2006), *Citizens at the Centre: Deliberative Participation in Healthcare Decisions*, Policy Press.

Dickenson, D. (2013), *Me Medicine vs. We Medicine: Reclaiming Biotechnology for the Common Good*, Columbia University Press.

Epstein, S. (1996), *Impure Science: AIDS, Activism, and the Politics of Knowledge*, University of California Press.

Galasso, I., and Geiger, S. (2021), Health Datafication and Justice. *Data Justice Conference*, May 25–28, Cardiff.

Geiger, H. J. (2017), The Political Future of Social Medicine: Reflections on Physicians as Activists. *Academic Medicine*, 92:3, 282–4.

Geiger, S. (2020), *Why We Need to Talk about Access Now!* MISFIRES Blogpost, October. Available at: https://misfires.ucd.ie/blogs/.

Geiger, S., and Gross, N. (2018), Market Failures and Market Framings: Can a Market Be Transformed from the Inside? *Organization Studies*, 39:10, 1357–76.

Geiger, S., and Gross, N. (2021), A tidal wave of inevitable data? Assetization in the consumer genomics testing industry. *Business & Society* 6:3, 614–49.

Geiger, S., Harrison, D., Kjellberg, H., and Mallard, A. (eds) (2014), *Concerned Markets: Economic Ordering for Multiple Values*, Edward Elgar Publishing.

Hoeyer, K., Bauer, S., and Pickersgill, M. (2019), Datafication and Accountability in Public Health: Introduction to a Special Issue. *Social Studies of Science*, 49:4, 459–75.

Hogle, L. F. (2016), Data-Intensive Resourcing in Healthcare, *BioSocieties*, 11:3, 372–93. doi:10.1057/s41292-016-0004-5.

Hummel, P., and Braun, M. (2020), Just Data? Solidarity and Justice in Data-Driven Medicine. *Life Sciences, Society and Policy*, 16:8.

Ismail, F., and Kamat, S. (2018), NGOs, Social Movements and the Neoliberal State: Incorporation, Reinvention, Critique, *Critical Sociology*, 44:4–5, 569–77.

Jasanoff, S. (ed.) (2004), *States of Knowledge: The Co-production of Science and the Social Order*, Routledge.

Love, J. (2020), The Use and Abuse of the Phrase "Global Public Good." Available at: https://developingeconomics.org/2020/07/16/the-use-and-abuse-of-the-phrase-global-public-good/.

Lowry, R. (2020), Only the "Crooks" of the Pharmaceutical Industry Can Save Us Now, *Politico Magazine*, March 18. Available at: https://www.politico.com/news/magazine/2020/03/18/only-the-crooks-of-the-pharmaceutical-industry-can-save-us-now-136255.

Martin, B. (2007), Activism, Social and Political, in G. L. Anderson and K. G. Herr (eds) *Encyclopedia of Activism and Social Justice*, Sage, 20–7.

Mason, K., and Araujo, L. (2020), Implementing Marketization in Public Healthcare Systems: Performing Reform in the English National Health Service, *British Journal of Management*. https://doi.org/10.1111/1467-8551.12417.

Matthews, D. (2020), Coronavirus: How Countries Aim to Get the Vaccine First by Cutting Opaque Supply Deals. *The Conversation*. Available at: https://theconversation.com/coronavirus-how-countries-aim-to-get-the-vaccine-first-by-cutting-opaque-supply-deals-143,366.

McLoughlin, I. P., Garrety, K., and Wilson, R. (2017), *The Digitalization of Healthcare: Electronic Records and the Disruption of Moral Orders*, Oxford University Press.

Mold, A. (2015), *Making the Patient-Consumer: Patient Organisations and Health Consumerism in Britain*, Manchester University Press.

Mountford, N., and Geiger, S. (2021), The Outside of Markets and the Upside of Fields: Foundational Concepts and a Research Agenda. *Academy of Marketing Science Review*.

Nik-Khah, E. (2018), Genomics and the Political Economy of Medicine, in S. Gibbon, B. Prainsack, S. Hilgartner, and J. Lamoreaux (eds) *Routledge Handbook of Genomics, Health and Society*, Routledge, 90–8.

Ostrom, V., and Ostrom, E. (2015), Public Goods and Public Choices, in D. H. Cole and M. D. McGinnis (eds) *Elinor Ostrom and the Bloomington School of Political Economy*, Lexington Books, 3–36.

Powles, J., and Hodson, H. (2017), Google DeepMind and Healthcare in an Age of Algorithms, *Health Technologies*, 7, 351–67.

Prainsack, B. (2018), The "We" in the "Me" Solidarity and Health Care in the Era of Personalized Medicine, *Science, Technology, and Human Values*, 43:1, 21–44.

Prainsack, B. (2019), Logged Out: Ownership, Exclusion and Public Value in the Digital Data and Information Commons, *Big Data and Society*, 6:1, 1–15.

Puig de la Bellacasa, M. (2017), *Matters of care: speculative ethics in more than human worlds, Posthumanities*, Minnesota: University of Minnesota Press.

Rabeharisoa, V. (2003), The Struggle against Neuromuscular Diseases in France and the Emergence of the "Partnership Model" of Patient Organisation, *Social Science and Medicine*, 57:11, 2127–36.

Rabeharisoa, V., Moreira, T., and Akrich, M. (2014), Evidence-Based Activism: Patients', Users' and Activists' Groups in Knowledge Society, *BioSocieties*, 9:2, 111–28.

Roelvink, G. (2015), *Making Other Worlds Possible: Performing Diverse Economies*, University of Minnesota Press.

Rose, N., and Novas, C. (2005), Biological Citizenship, in A. Ong and S. Collier (eds) *Global Assemblages: Technology, Politics, and Ethics as Anthropological Problems*, Blackwell, 439–63.

Samuelson, P. A. (1954), The Pure Theory of Public Expenditure, *Review of Economics and Statistics*, 387–9.

Scholz, M., and Smith, N. C. (2020), In the Face of a Pandemic, Can Pharma Shift Gears? *MIT Sloan Management Review*. Available at: https://sloanreview.mit.edu/article/in-the-face-of-a-pandemic-can-pharma-shift-gears/.

Sharon, T. (2018), When Digital Health Meets Digital Capitalism, How Many Common Goods Are at Stake? *Big Data and Society*, 5:2, 1–12.

Stendahl, E., and Geiger, S. (2020), Does Collective Always Mean Cohesive? Collective Institutional Entrepreneurship and Radical Flanks, *Academy of Management Proceedings*, 1.

Wehling, P., Viehöver, W., and Koenen, S. (eds) (2014), *The Public Shaping of Medical Research: Patient Associations, Health Movements and Biomedicine*, Routledge.

White House (2015), Fact Sheet: Precedent Obama's Precision Medicine Initiative. Available at: https://obamawhitehouse.archives.gov/the-press-office/2015/01/30/fact-sheet-president-obama-s-precision-medicine-initiative.

Widdows, H., and Cordell, S. (2011), Why Communities and Their Goods Matter: Illustrated with the Example of Biobanks, *Public Health Ethics*, 4:1, 14–25.

Woodhouse, E., Hess. D., Breyman, S., and Martin, B. (2002), Science Studies and Activism: Possibilities and Problems for Reconstructivist Agendas, *Social Studies of Science*, 32:2, 297–319.

Zuiderent-Jerak, T. (2009), Competition in the Wild: Reconfiguring Healthcare Markets, *Social Studies of Science*, 39:5, 765–92.

2

Preventing "Exit," Eliciting "Voice"

Patient, Participant, and Public Involvement as Invited Activism in Precision Medicine and Genomics Initiatives

Ilaria Galasso and Susi Geiger

Introduction

Over the decades, we have seen many and diverse expressions of healthcare activism, some of which are scrutinized in other chapters of this book. Especially when their own or loved ones' health is at stake or jeopardized by contentious commercial, medical, or regulatory practices, people often mobilize and/or publicly articulate their interests to ensure they are taken into account. While activism may not always be comfortable to public or private healthcare organizations, the contributions of this book demonstrate that it is a vital mechanism for these institutions to consider the overflows, oversights, and invisible effects arising from their actions and decisions. This chapter considers how organizations may react if there is a *lack of* such voices and thus no opportunity to learn from those affected by an organization's decisions and practices. By grounding ourselves on Albert Hirschman's (1970) "exit, voice and loyalty" framework, we argue that the fervent activism we see around access to healthcare therapies and services, described in several other chapters of this book, is *not* as often directed at concerns around sharing data for medical research. We particularly focus on this absence in the case of genomics and more generally of precision medicine initiatives, which have exponentially grown in significance and in financial investment as a proportion of overall medical research. Participation by individuals in such initiatives by sharing their data is, we argue, a peculiar case in the healthcare domain. Health and, derivatively, healthcare, as extensively elaborated by the political philosopher Norman Daniels (see for example Daniels 1981, 1985, 2008, 2017) are quite literally vital to an individual given the essential contribution they make to the opportunities people can exercise in their lives. Accordingly, much

Ilaria Galasso and Susi Geiger, *Preventing "Exit," Eliciting "Voice": Patient, Participant, and Public Involvement as Invited Activism in Precision Medicine and Genomics Initiatives* In: *Healthcare Activism: Markets, Morals, and the Collective Good*. Edited by: Susi Geiger, Oxford University Press. © Ilaria Galasso and Susi Geiger 2021.
DOI: 10.1093/oso/9780198865223.003.0002

activism is aimed at widening access and participation options. By contrast, the benefits deriving from sharing data with precision medicine and genomics initiatives are usually very long term and often directed at future populations rather than those who decide to share their data. If there are concerns about any aspects of sharing data, then people might find it easier to simply not participate in these initiatives than to articulate their concerns.

In this chapter, we thus explore the power of the voices described in the upcoming chapters of this book through a counterfactual: namely the mechanisms that organizations have to implement to learn from participants, patients, and the wider public if voice is absent—mechanisms that we call "invited activism." Echoing the concept of "invited space" for participation (Cornwall 2002; Bucchi and Neresini 2008; Pratt 2018), we define invited activism as those voices that do not arise spontaneously among concerned actors, but that are initiated by organizations to make up for the lack of "spontaneous" activism and as opportunities for institutional learning. In particular, we scrutinize how this "invited activism" has developed around data-sharing programs for medical research in general and genomics initiatives more specifically, and how it became epitomized in these spaces as public and patient involvement (PPI) practices.

The German economist Albert Otto Hirschman (1970) distinguishes two essential reaction mechanisms related to dissatisfaction: exit (that is, opting out from an "objectionable state of affairs") and voice (that is, interest articulation to try to change that "state of affairs"). Hirschman's notion of voice is very closely related to the concept of *activism*, the core object of the analyses in this volume, which might be understood as a particular instance of voice. The current book volume offers an array of cases and examples where voice is mobilized and exercised in relation to healthcare issues and institutions, and many chapters also chart how said institutions learn from such exercise of voice.

According to Hirschman's framework, in many situations the relative ease of exit tends to "drive out" voice, while conversely voice is pushed to the surface when exit is unavailable. From this perspective, voluntary data sharing for medical research and access to medical care can arguably be situated at opposite ends of the spectrum in terms of reaction mechanisms. In a healthcare context, *exit is often not an option at all.* To the contrary, voice is typically directed at gaining or improving access to a service or a medical product in the first place—these are the "health access movements" (Brown and Zavestoski 2004), one of which Moran and Mountford describe in their chapter. By contrast, it is arguably almost too easy to opt out from voluntary data sharing

30   PREVENTING "EXIT," ELICITING "VOICE"

for future-oriented medical research, and this ease, according to Hirschman, *discourages* interest articulation.

By revisiting Hirschman's classic analysis on exit and voice, we argue that in principle, when the perceived or real "costs" related to sharing personal genetic information are not acceptable, the exit (or opt-out) option prevails over voice. On the other hand, we argue that involvement practices made available by precision medicine initiatives can be understood as institutional attempts to increase voice and therefore as "invited activism": facilitation to articulate interests in order to provide a possible alternative to opting out and a feedback mechanism around (potential) participants' concerns. We discuss the implications of PPI in data-sharing initiatives as invited activism, and we conclude by discussing its instrumental value by critically distinguishing between *public* involvement, *participant* involvement, and *patient* involvement as subcategories of invited activism. We finally interrogate the limits of voice in this invited format in the context of genomics initiatives.

This chapter focuses on participation in genomics initiatives in many senses: from mere data sharing to active roles in research programs' governance. In order to avoid ambiguities, we follow Woolley and colleagues' (2016) terminological distinction between *participation, engagement*, and *involvement*. We thus refer to "participation" as merely acting as "human subjects" or, more specifically in our case, sharing one's data. Consistently, by *participants* in genomics initiatives, we refer to individuals who share their data with those initiatives, without implying any further active role for them. To refer to more active forms of "participation," we use the term *engagement*, in the sense of communication with the public about the purpose or aims of the research, and the term *involvement* to describe situations in which "members of the public have an active role in the planning and conduct of the research itself, even to the level of choosing the scientific questions to be addressed" (2016, 18). It is in this latter sense that PPI is scrutinized in this chapter. The "participatory medicine" approach, as we explore it here, is the tendency to encompass these three levels of participation: to ultimately promote research participants from mere human subjects to proper research "partners," fully informed on, and fully informative for, an organization's research agenda.

This is a conceptual chapter. Our initial argument—the general failure of concerned actors to voice *spontaneously* around voluntary data sharing for future-oriented medical research—is not developed inductively. As per the notorious "problem of induction" (Henderson 2018), empirical research is problematic around arguing that something is *not* (or is scarcely) there. This argument is mainly developed *deductively*, through the application of

Hirschman's theoretical framework to the medical research domain. At the same time, this theoretical deduction is, if not validated, at least not invalidated by observations. As a matter of fact, the applicability and the application of Hirschman's theoretical framework to medical research, as well as all the subsequent implications here discussed—in particular our central argument of PPI as "invited activism" to compensate for the lack of "spontaneous" voicing—are grounded on years of research, observations, and fieldwork around precision medicine initiatives and their PPI practices. Galasso, in her doctoral research, analyzed in depth the promises, the expectations, and the concerns around the two precision medicine projects here referred to—Genomics England and the All of Us Research Program—through document and discourse analysis, qualitative interviews with key actors in the projects' governance and in the debates around them, and through direct experience of PPI gained by participating in consultation practices open to the general public (Galasso 2018). Together, Galasso and Geiger, as part of the European Research Council-funded project "MISFIRES and Market Innovation," (grant agreement No. 771217) have analyzed the PPI practices implemented in the context of genomics and precision medicine initiatives in a range of cases by interviewing project staff engaged with participant representatives, and in some cases participant representatives themselves. Although this chapter is not aimed at presenting the results of this empirical research, those results, as well as the authors' broader experience around precision medicine research initiatives, offer indirect background for our conceptual claims.

This chapter aims to contribute to this volume in two ways: (1) we aim to provide further cause for reflection around the key role of activism in healthcare by scrutinizing the "participatory turn" as an institutional endeavor to expand voice; and (2) we aim to provide insights into the diversity of voice articulation in the health domain and on its diverse roles, by focusing on the implications of the invited nature of PPI as opposed to other forms of voice analyzed in this volume. We hope that contrasting our arguments with the other cases in this book will contribute to the critical analysis of the transformative role of activism in general, and of the potential and limits of invited activism and of participatory medicine in particular.

In Section 1, we describe contemporary medicine, embodied by precision medicine, as essentially data-fed, and reflect on the potential benefits and the costs related to sharing one's data, and in particular genetic data, as an intrinsic part of precision medicine—bringing together two of the core dynamics described in Geiger's introductory chapter: personalization and datafication. In Section 2 we discuss the individual choice of opting out from these initiatives or of articulating discontent, as framed by Albert Hirschman in terms of "exit" versus "voice." In Section 3 we critically discuss the rise of participatory medicine and of PPI practices as "invited activism" in genomics initiatives. Finally, in Section 4 we lay the ground to scrutinize invited activism in comparison with other forms of healthcare activism.

1. Sharing (Genetic Data) in Contemporary Medicine: "Benefits" and "Costs"

1.1 Contemporary Medicine: Inclusive, Precise, Data-Fed

If medical knowledge and practice have always been grounded on comparative observations of similarities and differences in health and disease states—this is actually the principle of epidemiology itself—contemporary medical research facilitates and relies on these comparisons at an unprecedented scale. Cheaper, more powerful, and more widespread technologies for data collection and processing allow scaling up from molecular, to individual, to population levels and all the way down again to understand and possibly intervene in the development of health and disease conditions with unprecedented precision: this is exactly the precision boasted by the emerging medical approach called "precision medicine."

Precision medicine, a concept that does not equate to, but substantially overlaps with the notion of "personalized medicine" (several scholars analyzed the relationship between these terms, see for instance Juengst et al. 2016 and Chan and Erikainen 2018), is generally defined as "prevention and treatment strategies that take individual variability into account" (Collins and Varmus 2015, 793). In precision medicine, this is typically done by following an essentially *data-driven* approach (Hogle 2016): individual data are analyzed against those of the general population. Consequently, in this framework, it is vital that truly population-wide data are available: the more massive and the more diverse the dataset, the better. Accordingly, the cutting-edge frontiers of precision in medicine are pursued by implementing huge national and international research cohort programs: Genomics England in the United Kingdom, the All of Us Research Program in the United States, GenomeAsia 100K, the forthcoming 1 + Million Genomes initiative in the European Union, and Three Million African Genomes on the African continent are some leading examples.

Participating in precision medicine research initiatives may involve sharing several different kinds of data: genetic data by providing specimens, lifestyle or demographic data by filling in surveys, biometric data by undergoing physical measurements, physiological and lifestyle data by providing access to wearable devices, medical history data by sharing electronic health records...In fact it is the combination of these different kinds of data that is supposed to foster "precision." Although the argument developed in this chapter around opting out prevailing over voicing in case of dissatisfaction is in principle applicable to all these types of data—actually, it is applicable to any sort of data one can voluntary share without expecting direct benefits—the main focus in this chapter is *genetic* data. Precision medicine research initiatives are very diverse, and different kinds of data are differently emphasized to the extent that providing a univocal definition of "precision medicine" may be challenging (Galasso 2018). Nonetheless, for most initiatives identified as precision medicine, genetic data play a preeminent role: genetic predispositions and the genetic components of diseases, although at interplay with other factors ranging from lifestyle to social and environmental determinants, are assumed to play a key role in the pursuit of precision in medicine. Accordingly, performing massive whole genome sequencing is considered the most promising frontier for the understanding, the prevention, and the treatment of a broad range of adverse health conditions.

1.2 Sharing Genetic Data: Individual and Social Benefits

In principle, by sharing their (genetic) data with genomics initiatives, individuals could benefit both themselves and others (Tutton and Prainsack 2011). Participants could gain benefits themselves because, by receiving their own genetic information back—as offered by most precision medicine research initiatives—they learn about their specific conditions and predispositions. They could benefit others by contributing to the advancement of medical research itself, as their genetic data provide the basis of comparison for understanding the key factors for specific disease onset and treatment.

The promise of individual benefits is particularly significant for genetic disease patients (including cancer and many rare disease patients): participation may sometimes lead to a long-awaited diagnosis and/or point to appropriate treatment; in other cases a mutation can be identified that can help with decisions about the most effective therapy, as in the famous case of trastuzumab (better known under its brand name Herceptin), a monoclonal

34 PREVENTING "EXIT," ELICITING "VOICE"

antibody specifically effective for treating HER2 positive breast cancer (www. drugs.com/mtm/trastuzumab.html). Beyond such special cases, genomics initiatives mainly provide research inputs about associations between genetic traits, external factors, and different disease onsets and responses to treatments, which will help prevent or better understand *future* cases rather than diagnosing or treating those patients who provided the data. Moreover, most genomics initiatives request data not only from genetic disease patients, but from the general population in order to better understand associations and efficient interventions (among those mentioned in Section 1.1, Genomics England is the only exception). In those cases, discourses mostly focus around the notion of *empowerment* (for a critical analysis of empowerment in precision medicine see Prainsack 2017): individuals are promised insights into their overall predispositions and genetic risks, which may aid them in managing their own health and regulating their lifestyle accordingly. However, the concrete advantages are in most cases limited, as structural means or social support are also needed for the individual to actually put informed choices into practice (Egger and Swinburn 1997; Juengst et al. 2016; Chiapperino and Testa 2016; Prainsack 2017), and as information related to risk and predisposition are questioned as not always reliable, significant, or actionable (Buchanan et al. 2006; Millikan 2006; Prainsack et al. 2008; Rose 2013; Tutton 2014; Hogle 2016; Prainsack 2017).

To sum up, it is unlikely that individuals will derive direct benefits from sharing genetic data, with the exception of some particular cases among genetic disease patients. The benefits from genetic data sharing, as for most kinds of medical research and epidemiological studies, are generally only materialized in the long term and not necessarily to the direct advantage of those who shared.

1.3 The Costs of Sharing Genetic Data

Despite the potential individual, communal, and societal advantages gained from participating in genomics initiatives, sharing one's genetic data is not costless. These costs may not be financial—while the consumer costs for sequencing charged by private consumers genomics companies start from less than one hundred euros, participation in national cohorts is generally free, and some even offer nominal compensation to cover travel expenses (in the case of All of Us, twenty-five US dollars). The costs of participating in genetics initiatives—whether potential, perceived, or real—are related to the many remaining uncertainties, most evidently among them loss of privacy and control over one's own genetic data.

Given the exceptional sensitivity of the data involved, concerns over data protection are often central in decisions to participate in genomics research initiatives (Middleton et al. 2019). Among other things, genetic data contain information that is unknown to the data-sharing individuals themselves. Moreover, this information relates not only to the sharer, but also to their relatives. Who has access to these data, and how these data are used now and in the future, are major concerns around genomics initiatives. Apart from concerns over political surveillance, other potential considerations of data use and misuse range from commercialization by private entities to new forms of discrimination. The most serious of these concerns have been advanced in terms of "genetic discrimination" in case genetic information becomes accessible to insurance companies or to employers (Billings et al. 1992; Kitcher 1996; Clayton 2003; Wolf 2005; Epstein 2007; Van Hoyweghen 2007).

It is important to note that many people might not be aware of the risks mentioned above, for instance that such a thing as "genetic discrimination" exists. Or, even if this is specified in consent forms, they might not realize that there is a risk for example that third parties might access their genetic data, or that their data sharing might have consequences for their family members as well. By contrast, some people might be concerned about less realistic risks, such as being cloned, or having their DNA copied and planted on the scene of a crime (Middleton et al. 2019).

1.4 Called upon for Sharing Data: Weighing Up Costs and Benefits

In the case of large-scale genomics initiatives, whatever the perceived costs and benefits, virtually every individual is invited to share their genetic data. Weighing up the costs and benefits of this data volunteering leaves individuals with a stark choice: if they do not share their genetic data for sequencing, individuals will miss out on information about themselves, which will remain invisible. If individuals want their genetic information to be visible to themselves, they have to share it with others. The same holds if they are moved by solidaristic or altruistic motivations about "donating" their genomic information to benefit their community or the broad society by contributing to medical research: they can do so only by incurring the risks related to genetic information disclosure. For patients suffering from genetic diseases, this

36 PREVENTING "EXIT," ELICITING "VOICE"

equation might be a simple one: bearing the "cost" of the disease they hope to treat might well exceed the risk of losing privacy and control over their data, or even the more remote risks of future surveillance or discrimination. For the general public, however, the risk–benefit balance might not always be so straightforward.

In this chapter, we analyze the dynamics developing around the *refusal* of incurring the costs and risks of data sharing. We acknowledge that if some people decide not to participate in genomics initiatives, this is not always necessarily because of the perceived "costs," however broadly framed. Many people may never be reached by an invitation to participate, may not care, may for a variety of reasons deliberately not want to know the information embedded in their genomes, may not wish to contribute to medical research, or may not believe their contribution would bring significant benefits to their community or to society. However, in our analysis, we focus on what we call the "opt-outs"—those people who, in principle, would be interested in participating in genomics initiatives, but are held back or hesitant because of the "costs."

2. Exit, Opt-Out, and Voice in Genomics Initiatives

2.1 Hirschman's Framework

As we scrutinize the dynamics around opting out of participation in genomics initiatives, we ground our argument on Albert Otto Hirschman's classic book *Exit, Voice and Loyalty* (1970). Hirschman argues that there are essentially two *reaction mechanisms* pursued by discontented customers or members of an organization—*exit* and *voice*—with possible combinations of these two. In general terms, through exit, customers leave or opt out of the organization that dissatisfies them; in the opposite case, through voice, as in the activist movements analyzed in this volume, they "attempt to change" what dissatisfies them by expressing their discontent to the organization itself and hope that it will learn.

Hirschman's examples range from consumer firms to parties and nation states and do not explicitly refer to the domain of health, healthcare, or health data sharing. However, Hirschman's framework is very broadly relevant to any instance of participation as voluntary activity (Kelty et al. 2015): it is virtually applicable to any situation in which there is a choice about being part of, subscribing to, or accessing, any sort of transaction, service, organization, group, institution, or initiative, provided it is possible to opt out and to articulate discontent. Concerning the medical domain, Hirschman's analysis has been applied to patients' reactions to discontent toward healthcare providers (Annas 1997; Brüggemann 2017) or health systems (Ippolito et al. 2013). In relation to genetic testing specifically, Hirschman's work has been used to advocate for the development of proper consultation instead of a binary opt-in/opt-out choice (Benschop et al. 2003), and for public consultation around genomic testing regulations (De Vries and Horstman 2008).

In line with these works, we think through people's reaction mechanisms when there is discontent about the conditions for sharing genetic data for medical research. In particular we focus on the importance of voice in a field that is characterized by doubts and uncertainties (Benschop et al. 2003). We interrogate how genomics and precision medicine initiatives deal with the problem that in the context of genetic testing, "informative voice" tends to be drowned out by "silent and uninformative participation or silent and uninformative exit" (2003, 147), or in other words, that "the potential of voice to improve practices is clearly under-used" (De Vries and Horstman 2008, 185). Much has changed in the years since these two studies applying Hirschman's framework in the domain of genetic testing were written: on the one hand genomics initiatives have reached unprecedented spread and preeminence, making a renewed scrutiny of the reaction mechanisms of "exit" and "voice" in the genomics context necessary. On the other hand, over the past decade medical research has experienced a "participatory turn," giving "voice" a central role, actualized most prominently in the implementation of PPI practices. This participatory turn is particularly evident around genomics initiatives where "the advantages of voice as a feedback mechanism" (De Vries and Horstman 2008, 182) have gained a renewed institutional recognition.

The centrality of voice in current genomics initiatives' practices is the object of Section 3. In this section, we apply the framework developed by Hirschman to contemporary genomics initiatives.

2.2 Exit: Withdrawing versus Opting Out

With regard to the first of Hirschman's two options, namely exit, we pursue a broad interpretation of the notion of exit, one that extends the notion from former customers or participants to what we call opt-outs, that is people who are *invited* to be participants in precision medicine initiatives but who have not participated before. Exit in the narrow sense of withdrawal of former participants may be questioned as somehow incomplete in the context of genetic data sharing: although withdrawal generally guarantees destruction of the provided specimens and prohibition for any further use of those data, this does generally not apply to data already used, and in any case nothing can be done about information that has already circulated. As a consequence, some costs and benefits cannot be reversed through exit: the benefit of becoming aware of one's own genomic information is received as soon as information is delivered and cannot be withdrawn, while the costs are not (entirely) canceled out either as previously disclosed information can never be really destroyed.

Given the peculiarity of the exit-as-withdrawal option in the genomics domain, in our analysis we compare voice with opt-out or non-participation, as *the only way to really exit from a genomics initiative is not entering at all*. We argue that Hirschman's analysis remains applicable to our argument if we shift the reaction mechanisms to an earlier stage, namely, when the patient or citizen still has to decide whether becoming a data donor at all: it is (only) at this stage, through opt-out, that in the case of genomics initiatives invited participants can truly "escape from an objectionable state of affairs" (Hirschman 1970, 30).

In the case of genomics initiatives, the opt-out option generates a no-win situation: individuals opting out lose the opportunity to access (and possibly be empowered by) their own genomic information; the genomics initiative loses future profits and possibly breadth of research applicability; and society and specific communities lose benefits possibly deriving from future health-care design and services. As a matter of fact, precision medicine and data-fed research in general is a prototypical case in which "exit [opt-out] of a member leads to further deterioration in the quality of the organization's output" (Hirschman 1970, 101), as far as this research grounds its "precision" and applicability on massive and diverse data. An extreme case of mass opt-outs (refusal to participate) could signal the potential collapse of data-driven initiatives. The exit option, then, is *a multi-edged failure* in the context of genomics initiatives. Nonetheless, in line with Hirschman's analysis, the opt-out option is likely the prevalent reaction mechanism in the context of dissatisfaction or suspicion around genomics initiatives. Opt-out is a straight-forward action for potential participants: it only requires to ignore advertise-ments or invitations to share data, and it even avoids the mundane "costs" of participation, related for example to getting in touch with the initiative, going through the informed consent process, undergoing potential physical tests, and giving samples. Thus, consistent with Hirschman's intuition that "easy exit" drives out voice, people who are invited to participate in precision medicine initiatives and are unhappy with the conditions provided can simply ignore the invitation and are very unlikely to articulate their discontent or negotiate different conditions.

Importantly, this reflection does not imply that all potential participants will choose to exit: some will share their genetic data because of a variety of reasons that can range from expected empowerment to mere curiosity (Geiger and Gross 2021); some will still share their data out of loyalty and solidarity (despite some concerns we are going to discuss), in view of the benefits they expect genomics initiatives might provide to society; others, because they have not considered the costs or risks of participation. Many individuals, despite the possible concerns discussed, are happy enough with the conditions, as demonstrated by the fact that millions of individuals globally have agreed to share their genomic data both with private companies and with national programs. Nonetheless, if our analysis is correct, dissatisfied individuals are likely to simply opt out, without ever articulating why they chose to do so, depriving the organizations in question of a vital learning mechanism.

2.3 Voice: Political and Costly

In Hirschman's analysis, voice is "political action par excellence" (1970, 16). Similar to activism, which might be understood as a particular instance of it, voice "can be graduated, all the way from faint grumbling to violent protest" (1970, 16), but it always implies clear "interest articulation": in contrast to exit, voice is defined

> as any attempt at all to change, rather than to escape from, an objectionable state of affairs, whether through individual or collective petition to the management directly in charge, through appeal to a higher authority with the intention of forcing a change in management, or through various types of actions and protests, including those that are meant to mobilize public opinion. (1970, 30)

A crucial point emphasized by Hirschman is that, in general, when the exit (or opt-out) option is available and easy to use, it "drives out" voice. The argument proceeds by noting that "in comparison to the exit option, voice is costly" to the individual. As a matter of fact, "buyers of a product or members of an organization spend time and money in the attempt to achieve changes in the policies and practices of the firm from which they buy or of the organization to which they belong." Moreover, "voice will depend also on the willingness to take the chances of the voice option as against the certainty of the exit option" (1970, 40).

The consequence of people simply opting out without making themselves heard engenders, in line with Hirschman's argument, institutional entropy: there is no way for the organization to know whether individuals are not sharing their data because of lack of interest or information or because they have any specific concern about the procedures or the conditions, what these concerns are, and how they could be addressed (Van Hoyweghen 2007; Middleton et al. 2018).

With this argument, we claim that discontented potential participants generally fail to articulate their dissatisfaction, but with this we do *not* want to give the misleading idea that no concerns and no requests at all are ever articulated around the way genetic data are managed by genomics initiatives. On the contrary, regulators, ethicists, and some non-governmental organizations are very active on that front—counterinstitutional voice, so to speak, does exist, but it is usually the voice of the expert and not of the users themselves. Also, in line with our characterization of having shared genetic data as creating a "no-exit situation" to the extent that full withdrawal cannot be guaranteed, individual or public voice is most likely to take place after "the damage is done," for instance when conditions change after data have already been shared, such as when the genomics initiative is acquired by or has partnered with another company, or when data are used beyond participants' consent. Famous historical and contemporary examples include the use and publication of Henrietta Lacks' genome (Skloot 2010), the accusation to the Wellcome Trust Sanger Institute of commercialization plans for African DNA (Stokstad 2019), the use of Havasupai Indians' genomes for broader research than initially understood (Harmon 2010), and the acquisition of the Ogliastra people's genomes by an English company (Manis 2018). In these cases, although often "partial exit" is pursued by withdrawing, as discussed, total exit is not possible. Consequently, voice generally finds some space in these contexts, contrary to cases of discontent when opt-out is still available.

2.4 Loyalty: Participating for the Sake of Public Good?

In Hirschman's analysis, the binary distinction between exit and voice is elaborated in connection with a third concept, which may also be relevant in the context of genomics initiatives: *loyalty*. Hirschman defines loyalty as "a generalized concept of penalty for exit" (1970, 98), which occurs when for some reason consumers/members do not want to quit a service that they are dissatisfied with. Whatever the reasons are, they are very important in Hirschman's analysis insofar as the derived loyalty "helps to redress the balance by raising the cost of exit."

According to Hirschman, "loyalist behavior" typically arises, among other scenarios, in the context of "public goods." He defines public goods as "goods which are consumed by all those who are members of a given community, country, or geographical area in such a manner that consumption or use by one member does not detract from consumption or use by another" (1970, 101). Public health features among the standard examples of public goods provided by Hirschman himself. Thus, as far as they are contributing to the general advancement of healthcare, medical research projects in general and genomics initiatives in particular might be considered "organizations producing public goods." As a consequence, participating (or not) in these initiatives means participating (or not) in the production of a public good. Awareness of this point is deeply connected to the altruistic motivations for sharing data for medical/genomics research discussed above and could in principle encourage data sharing even when there is (some) dissatisfaction around the initiative's terms and conditions.

On the other hand, and potentially thwarting the "public good" argument (as well as those voices calling for an obligation to participate in medical research, among others: Petersen and Lupton 1996; Chadwick and Berg 2001; Rhodes 2005, 2008, 2017; Schaefer et al. 2009; Faden et al. 2013) there is widespread concern that medical innovation might exacerbate existing healthcare inequalities by predominantly benefitting people who are already advantaged in the healthcare system, and this concern is especially emphasized in the context of precision medicine (Galasso 2018). The debate about the effects of precision medicine on healthcare costs and accessibility is an open one, and not one we are likely to solve in this chapter. In any case, those individuals who cannot access even basic healthcare will no doubt be similarly unable to access precision medicine treatments, both under private as well as public healthcare systems (Modi 2017). Thus, as long as they are not accessible by a (large) part of society, precision medicine benefits cannot be defined as "public" goods. Conversely, in some cases they risk being very exclusive and exclusionary goods. In such cases, as argued by Dickenson (2013), the premise of altruism and solidarity collapses in favor of a highly individualistic and entrepreneurial framework.

To summarize our argument thus far, health research and care generally are one of the few contexts in which exit is generally costlier than voice: given the essential relevance of health in terms of opportunities people can exercise

(Daniels 1981, 1985, 2008, 2017), while exit may theoretically be possible—in the sense that it is *possible* not to access therapies, or to accept that your disease is not recognized or addressed by research—it tends to be so costly to the individual that it cannot practically be considered as an option at all. Thus we argue that access to healthcare and inclusion in medical research, especially when there are direct individual health interests at stake, can be considered as no-exit situations. Consistent with Hirschman's thinking around no-exit situations, and as demonstrated across this book's pages, this makes voice the predominant reaction mechanism (although not availing of therapies for economic reasons is a widespread problem; Osservatorio Donazione Farmaci 2018).

The situation is very different in the case of sharing genetic data. Given, (1) Hirschman's argument on the prominence of exit over voice whenever exit is easily available, (2) the observed extreme ease of opt-out from genomics initiatives, and (3) the discussed potential inability of these initiatives to produce public goods and to foster loyalist behaviors to counterbalance exit; we conclude that exit (opt-out) is expected to be the prevalent reaction to dissatisfaction in the context of data sharing for future-oriented medical research, at the expense of interest articulation through voice.

3. Participatory Medicine

3.1 Switching from Exit to Voice

In Section 1, we discussed how large-scale and diverse participation in genomics initiatives (and more generally in medical research) is essential to guarantee the advancement and broad applicability of medical innovation. As long as opt-out appears the obvious option for dissatisfied potential participants, the applicability, inclusivity, and equitability of genomics research might be jeopardized. In parallel, massive opt-out also jeopardizes the goals and even the existence of the genomics initiatives themselves, as they ground their success on the results they can extrapolate and use from participants' data.

Against this scenario, it would be in the interest of all stakeholders to "redress the balance" and encourage voice over exit. According to Hirschman's analysis, the most straightforward way to do so is to eliminate the exit option, by creating a no-exit situation in which voice becomes the only option. This scenario—provided that it is desirable—is not possible in the case of genomics initiatives and of medical research, unless by repudiating all the ethical principles that have been established in the last century and fostering a society in which everyone is *forced* to share their genetic information. Another option, as discussed in Section 2, involves "raising the costs of exit" through loyalty by improving and expanding accessibility to forthcoming healthcare benefits as "public goods." However, as mentioned, as long as there is potential exclusivity of the goods produced by precision medicine initiatives, loyalty has limited applicability in this context.

If increasing loyalty or the cost of exit is not possible or is dismissed as an option, the only other way to "redress the balance" between exit/voice is, quite obviously, decreasing the cost of voice. Or, in other words, providing infrastructures and facilities to encourage interest articulation. In the words of Hirschman:

> The creation of effective new channels through which consumers can communicate their dissatisfaction holds one important lesson. While structural constraints (availability of close substitutes, number of buyers, durability and standardization of the article, and so forth) are of undoubted importance in determining the balance of exit and voice for individual commodities, the propensity to resort to the voice option depends also on the general readiness of a population to complain and on the *invention* of such institutions and mechanisms as can communicate complaints cheaply and effectively.
>
> (Hirschman 1970, 43, emphasis in the original text)

In contemporary medical research, the creation of "channels through which consumers can communicate their dissatisfaction" might be envisioned as embodied by the emerging framework of "participatory medicine." This model promotes a more extensive implementation of participation in medical research, also embracing what Woolley and colleagues (2016) refer to as *engagement* and *involvement*. Within this framework, citizens are invited to participate at many levels: not just to take part as human subjects, but also to be *engaged* in the research, in the sense of understanding the background, the purposes, and the utility of the research itself and their own roles in it, and even to be *involved* in decision making and priority setting.

Although not all genomics and precision medicine research studies—and certainly not all at the same level and in the same way—embrace a "participatory turn," perhaps unsurprisingly given our analysis thus far, this rhetoric has been heavily embraced in the context of those initiatives that entirely rely on massive and diverse voluntary participation in data sharing: "without patients contributing data, time, effort and self-care, current vision of

44 PREVENTING "EXIT," ELICITING "VOICE"

personalized medicine cannot be realized... it is not a coincidence that we see a renewed emphasis on patient participation at a time when medicine is particularly hungry for data and other contributions from us all" (Prainsack 2017, 11).

3.2 "Participants as Partners"

With the recurring motto of involving "participants as partners" (https://allofus.nih.gov), some of the main national precision medicine cohort studies have opened up several kinds of channels through which (potential) participants are facilitated to express their concerns and articulate their interests. All of Us in the US and Genomics England in the United Kingdom are especially active on that front: they have circulated surveys and "requests for information" to the general public, organized public dialogue, focus groups, panel discussions, and public events, made available (online and offline) forms for nominating diseases to be included in the research, and they have leaned on digital platforms allowing people to share their "ideas" about research priorities. Moreover, both All of Us and Genomics England have involved lay participants in their governance: both initiatives have "participant panels," which are composed of participant representatives and are to act as advisory bodies and be engaged with decision making across the initiatives.

In this framework, given the variety of "channels" provided to meet the preferences of everyone, voice becomes less "costly" and in fact is also supposed to be *easy*. Channels for voice are broadly advertised and made to be easily accessible. Voice still remains not completely costless, as certain skills, time, and energy are required to formulate interests or concerns. But these costs are no longer so disproportionate to the "free" exit option. The "invention of these channels" might, at least in principle, succeed in "redress[ing] the exit/voice balance" and "hav[ing] the members of the organization switch from exit to voice" (Hirschman 1970, 123).

3.3 "Voice from Within and Voice from Without": Patient, Participant, and Public Involvement

The specific "channels of voice" offered by precision medicine and genomics initiatives in alignment with the paradigm of "participatory medicine" might take on very different forms. Here we focus on one of the most relevant distinctions to our analysis on exit and voice: the channels for "voice from within," and the channels for "voice from without" (Hirschman 1970). In other words, we propose to analyze the significance and implications of offering and facilitating the opportunity for voice for those who *opted out* (have not participated in) vis-à-vis for those who have *opted into* genomics initiatives.

As seen, the practices made available in participatory medicine to extend the scope of participation are often addressed as PPI. However, scholars have urged to "split apart the familiar acronym, drawing a distinction between patient and public involvement, rather than treating PPI as a single practice," as "justification for involving the public differs in ethically significant ways from the justification for involving patients" (McCoy et al. 2019, 709). In this section we follow McCoy and colleagues' suggestion. In our case, as people who opt into precision medicine initiatives are not necessarily "patients" in the strict sense of the term, rather than only distinguishing between *public* and *patient* involvement, we suggest to add another term of distinction that, coincidentally, also starts with the letter P: *participant* involvement (we might talk of PPPI!). In our analysis, participants are all those individuals who opted into a precision medicine initiative with which they shared their data, irrespective of their clinical conditions. Consistently, participant involvement is defined as all those practices to articulate interests or concerns available to individuals who have shared their (genetic) data with the initiative at issue, or, in some specific cases, to their guardians or carers. In other words, the concept of participant involvement is applied to all those participatory practices that *exclude* those who opt out. Conversely, we define the public as all individuals belonging to a population, irrespective of whether they shared their (genetic) data or not. Consistently, we define public involvement as all those practices to articulate interests or concerns that are available to any individual in the population, *including* those who opt out. As for the definition of "patient," it is especially problematic in the context of genetic testing: virtually anyone can be included in this category, especially if *risk* of disease is included. To avoid ambiguities, in our analysis, we refer as "patients" to all those people who are addressed *because of* their clinical conditions (or, in some cases, their carers). In some cases, patient and participant involvement might coincide: this is the case of research initiatives only recruiting specific patients, as Genomics England does. However, most genomics initiatives invite the general population to share data, independent of their clinical conditions, and if there are no individuals specifically participating *as* patients, then there is no space for a proper patient involvement outside of participant involvement—unless specific events or forums are set up by specifically focusing on a given health condition.

The two precision medicine initiatives that we already mentioned as outstanding in terms of embracing the framework of "participatory medicine"— All of Us and Genomics England—involve the general public, participants, and patients in different ways (Galasso and Testa 2017; Galasso 2018). Genomics England is mostly, if not entirely, focused on patient/participant involvement (coinciding in this case, as all participants participate *in virtue of* their condition as patients): some *participant* representatives are included in the governance of the project, while the general public is generally addressed in terms of *engagement*, in the sense that diverse public events and dialogues are implemented to provide wide and deep understanding of the project, without including a proper involvement of the public for decision making. On the other hand, All of Us—which likewise involves some participant representative in the project governance—has also made available several practices for *public* involvement, such as digital platforms and online forms where virtually anyone in the world could provide comments and proposals on specified aspects of the project. All of Us, in comparison to Genomics England, provides space for a plurality of voices, but they offer poor transparency around the impact of those voices. This may undermine what, according to the analysis by Kelty and colleagues (2015), is one of the fundamental dimensions of "proper participation" as opposed to tokenism.

Where our analysis casts the facilitation of voice as a counterbalance to exit and as a feedback mechanism to avoid institutional entropy, public, patient, and participant involvement each have a deeply different meaning. *Public* involvement offers individuals an alternative to opt out. *Participant* involvement is, by definition, solely addressed to people who agreed to participate and aimed to either prevent their satisfaction from deteriorating or to improve it to build further barriers to exit. Providing participants with continuous opportunities to articulate their interests and concerns gives them the chance to express their dissatisfaction as soon as it emerges. Apart from that, participants, given their *insider* experience of the initiative and of the participatory process, become "experts" of sorts around data-sharing issues. As a consequence, participant involvement also embeds an important *instrumental* value to the organization (Sen 1999; McCoy et al. 2019): participants can provide valuable insights and suggestions to improve the organization and consequently the satisfaction of current or future participants. Beyond this insider's perspective, *patients*, be they participants or not, can provide unique expertise: they are proper experts, more than anyone else, on the conditions related to their own diseases. This unique expertise is explicitly valued for example in the context of the Genomics England Participant Panel. As discussed in Section 1, patients, in some cases, are those who can expect to benefit directly from participating in genomics initiatives, and thus they may balance risks and benefits in a different way to less directly concerned individuals. If patients decide not to participate in a genomics initiative, that decision is likely made on other grounds than simply opting for the ease of exit over voice. As a consequence, we can assume that patient involvement does not make a significant difference in terms of broadening participation. On the other hand, it is especially significant in terms of the *informativity* of voice (Benschop et al. 2003). Participant and patient involvement, especially if extended to the level of governance, would hence benefit both the quality and the democratic capacities of genomics initiatives and minimize opt-out.

In comparison with patient and participant involvement, in public involvement individuals may lack the direct internal expertise of the data-sharing initiative, but bring the perspective of those who are in principle interested in participating. By articulating their concerns, they can contribute to changing any conditions that would prevent them from doing so. Thus, public involvement has the advantage that it *directly* increases the likelihood of participation.

In summary, public, participant, and patient involvement may all contribute, in different and complementary ways, to more participant-friendly genomics initiatives, to broader and more diverse participation, and to more equitable healthcare benefits, and vice versa, in a virtuous circle. However, as will be briefly discussed in Section 4, it is essential that inclusivity and consistent power distribution are pursued in order to avoid a totally uninformative and even deceiving "presence without voice and voice without power" (Pratt 2018, 2).

4. Invited Activism

The picture that emerges by observing the forms of voice around voluntary data sharing for precision medicine, in line with Hirschman's analysis, is an almost exclusive preeminence of "invited spaces" over "created spaces" (Cornwell 2002; Pratt 2018) or, from another perspective, of "sponsored participation" over "spontaneous participation" (Bucchi and Neresini 2008). Two important implications emerge from this observation in the context of this book on activism in healthcare: first, that organizations have realized the unique importance of individual and collective voice for institutional learning and innovation, to the extent that the contemporary paradigm of participatory medicine can, at least in part, be understood as compensating for the lack of activism in certain areas, or at least as facilitating the expression of (patient) voice. And second, that despite these efforts, given this exclusively "invited" nature, quintessential differences exist between voice in the form of PPI/PPPI in data-sharing medical initiatives and healthcare activism in other contexts.

As Chapter 1 highlighted, definitions of activism are generally very broad, consistent with the variety of its forms and expressions. However, the distinctive feature of activism as commonly accepted is that "it assumes some intervention in the public domain *that goes beyond institutionally sanctioned... activities*" (Woodhouse et al. 2002, 313, emphasis added). As a consequence, "invited activism" is in fact an oxymoron, and we are quick to admit this fact. Participatory medicine, as promoted by the initiatives themselves, is institutionalized, and, as such, cannot, by definition, provide a valid substitute for activism. Participatory medicine is different from proper activism as it is "invited," "sponsored," initiated, mediated, and regulated by the institution itself towards which activism is supposed to be addressed. Thus, invited activism in the form of PPI/PPPI or other participatory mechanisms will always be incomplete.

The distinctively "invited" nature of involvement in participatory medicine may cause some concerns. Even more so than "spontaneous" activism, invited activism, as initiated and mediated by the very same initiative toward which it is directed, might privilege certain voices over others (in terms of "who" will take up the invitation and who will be heard), might highlight selective messages over those that are particularly unwelcome by the organization in question (in terms of how the voicing will be understood and taken up), and might shape what can and cannot be articulated (in terms of the forums and channels provided).

In more detail, a first concern is related to exclusiveness: in addition to the barriers related to the skills and means required for utilizing even the most accessible voice channels, the fact that these practices are "upon invitation" and that invitations might be explicitly or implicitly targeted or even intentionally exclusive, exacerbates the risk that patterns of exclusion might emerge around involvement practices (Galasso 2018; Pratt 2018; Prainsack 2019). This may prevent some groups from switching from exit to voice, and it may erase their interests and needs from the initiative's agenda setting, thus exacerbating existing disparities.

A second concern is related to effectiveness—whether these voice channels lead to improvements that take account of the interests and needs expressed through voice. As a matter of fact, voice, *per se*, does *not* guarantee change.

Voice is defined as the *attempt* to change (Hirschman 1970, 130), but it could be "mere 'blowing off steam'" (1970, 124), and similarly the space provided for voice could be just an instrument that "allows the powerholders to claim that all sides were considered, but makes it possible for only some of those sides to benefit" (Arnstein 1969, 216). In the case of participatory medicine, and of invited activism in general, effectiveness is all the more problematic as interest articulations are structured and channeled by "the powerholders" themselves (the initiative), through the channels and to the aims that they themselves established. Yet, even this "tokenistic" scenario may lead to positive consequences for the organization: voice could still, in principle, decrease the opt-out rate through the *illusion* of having the possibility to change the state of affairs, and thus foster the "shift from exit to voice." This would still enhance participation and data sharing in precision medicine initiatives and, as a consequence, enhance the robustness and applicability of research findings. However, tokenistic involvement would provide little or no benefit to the research setting, and it would potentially further stifle the likelihood of spontaneous or uninvited activism. In other words, tokenistic involvement would be to the short-term advantage of the genomics initiatives but likely lead to institutional entropy in the long run.

Analyses of participatory medicine need to take the distinctiveness of its invited nature into full account: unlike other manifestations of activism discussed in this book, in participatory medicine it is the "object of debate" itself that initiates voice, that establishes its purpose, that establishes who participate and how (Pratt 2018). Research on PPI/PPPI needs to interrogate the extent to which this inherent conflict of interest influences the instrumental value of participation, and the extent to which it risks, voluntarily or involuntarily, creating bias and barriers for other types of activism, for a more inclusive redistribution of power, and for proper democratic innovation.

Conclusion

In this chapter, we discussed the essential role of activism, as demonstrated by the strategies implemented by institutions to compensate for a lack of activism and to trigger voice when it is not initiated spontaneously. In particular, we have analyzed involvement practices embraced by precision medicine cohort programs as a remedy to the silent opt-out or non-participation of individuals from those medical research initiatives that are reliant on public participation. We have argued that participatory medicine can facilitate inclusive and diverse participation in these initiatives by (1) providing valid and easy voice alternatives to those who otherwise would just opt out (in the case of public involvement); and (2) ameliorating the participatory conditions by including the perspectives of those who experience the participatory process from the inside (patient and participant involvement). In other words, the promotion of voice is expected to bring two advantages: broadening participation (voice instead of exit) and improving the organization of participation and of the research (voice as feedback mechanism). In principle, by granting concerned actors the opportunity to express their concerns and interests, invited activism promises a more inclusive framework of medical innovation, aimed at the pursuit of the public good by taking into account the needs and interests of the public. However, we discussed some concerns jeopardizing such a positive outcome, which, as seen, are all the more relevant in the context of participatory medicine as a form of invited activism: as such, we argued it needs to be analyzed taking this distinctiveness into full account.

Contrasting our arguments with the other cases in this book provides scope for further analysis of the transformative role of activism in general, and on the potential and limits of invited activism and of participatory medicine in particular, in contrast with "spontaneous" activism. In line with our argument, activism, even when perceived as a nuisance, obstacle, or a momentary slowdown from the perspective of the institutions towards which it is addressed, provides a unique opportunity for feedback and for triggering and regulating innovation. Ultimately, this is to the advantage of a multiplicity of stakeholders, as demonstrated by the fact that when activism is missing some surrogates are implemented by the institutions and initiatives themselves.

As for the essentiality of the role of activism for innovation, further research may helpfully compare our setting with other cases where activism for whatever reason does not generally arise spontaneously, to observe how institutions respond to missing activism in other contexts. Likewise, research around other instantiations of invited spaces for participation would help provide further insights for the understanding of the role of activism itself.

Acknowledgments

The authors have received funding for writing this chapter from the European Research Council (ERC) under the European Union's Horizon 2020 research and innovation programme (grant agreement No. 771217).

References

Annas, G. J. (1997), Patients' Rights in Managed Care – Exit, Voice, and Choice, *The New England Journal of Medicine*, 337, 210–215.

Arnstein, S. R. (1969), A Ladder of Citizen Participation, *Journal of the American Planning Association*, 35:4, 216–24.

Benschop, R., Horstman, K., and Vos, R. (2003), Voice beyond Choice: Hesitant Voice in Public Debates about Genetics in Health Care, *Health Care Analysis*, 11:2, 141–50.

Billings, P. R., Kohn, M. A., de Cuevas, M., Beckwith, J., Alper, J. S., and Natowicz, M. R. (1992), Discrimination as a Consequence of Genetic Testing, *American Journal of Human Genetics*, 50:3, 476–82.

Brown, P., and Zavestoski, S. (2004), Social Movements in Health: An Introduction, *Sociology of Health and Illness*, 26:6, 679–94.

Brüggemann, A. J. (2017), Exploring Patient Strategies in Response to Untoward Healthcare Encounters, *Nursing Ethics*, 24:2, 190–7.

Bucchi, M., and Neresini, F. (2008), Science and Public Participation, in E. J. Hackett, O. Amsterdamska, M. Lynch, and J. Wajcman (eds) *The Handbook of Science and Technology Studies* (3rd edition), MIT Press.

Buchanan, A. V., Weiss, K. M., and Fullerton, S. M. (2006), Dissecting Complex Disease: the Quest for the Philosopher's Stone? *International Journal of Epidemiology*, 35, 562–71.

Chadwick, R., and Berg, K. (2001), Solidarity and Equity: New Ethical Frameworks for Genetic Databases, *Nature Reviews Genetics*, 2:4, 318–21.

Chan, S., and Erikainen, S. (2018), What's in a Name? The Politics of "Precision Medicine," *American Journal of Bioethics*, 18:4, 50–2.

Chiapperino, L., and Testa, G. (2016), The epigenomic self in personalized medicine: between responsibility and empowerment, *The Sociological Review Monographs*, 64:1, 203–20.

Clayton, E. W. (2003), Ethical, Legal, and Social Implications of Genomic Medicine, *The New England Journal of Medicine*, 349, 562–69.

Collins, F. S., and Varmus, H. (2015), A New Initiative on Precision Medicine, *The New England Journal of Medicine*, 372, 793–5.

Cornwall, A. (2002), Making Spaces, Changing Places: Situating Participation in Development, IDS Working Paper 170.

Daniels, N. (1981), Health Care Needs and Distributive Justice, *Philosophy and Public Affairs*, 10:2, 146–79.

Daniels, N. (1985), *Just Health Care*, New York: Cambridge University Press.

Daniels, N. (2008), *Just Health: Meeting Health Needs Fairly*, New York: Cambridge University Press.

Daniels, N. (2017), Justice and Access to Health Care, *Stanford Encyclopedia of Philosophy* (Winter Edition), Edward N. Zalta (ed.). Available at: https://plato.stanford.edu/entries/justice-healthcareaccess/#DoesJustRequUnivAcceHealCare.

De Vries, G., and Horstman, K. (2008), Learning from the Work that Links Laboratory to Society, in *Genetics from Laboratory to Society: Societal Learning as an Alternative to Regulation*, Palgrave Macmillan.

Dickenson, D. (2013), *Me Medicine vs. We Medicine: Reclaiming Biotechnology for the Common Good*, Columbia University Press.

Egger, G., and Swinburn, B. (1997), An 'Ecological' Approach to the Obesity Pandemic, *British Medical Journal*, 315:7106, 477.

Epstein, S. (2007), *Inclusion: The Politics of Difference in Medical Research*, University of Chicago Press.

Faden, R. R., Kass, N. E., Goodman, S. N., Pronovost, P., Tunis, S., and Beauchamp, T. L. (2013), An Ethics Framework for a Learning Health Care System: a Departure from Traditional Research Ethics and Clinical Ethics, *Hastings Center Report*, January-February 2013, 16-27.

Galasso, I. (2018), *Precision Medicine in Society: Promises, Expectations and Concerns around Social and Health Equity*, PhD Dissertation, European School of Molecular Medicine and University of Milan.

Galasso, I., and Testa, G. (2017), Citizen Science and Precision Medicine: A Route to Democracy in Health?, *Harvard Law/Petrie Flom Center Bill of Health Blog*. Available at: http://blogs.harvard.edu/billofhealth/2017/05/10/citizen-science-and-precision-medicine-a-route-to-democracy-in-health/.

Geiger, S., and Gross, N. (2021), A Tidal Wave of Inevitable Data? Assetization in the Consumer Genomics Testing Industry, *Business and Society*, 60:3, 614–49.

Harmon, A. (2010), Indian Tribe Wins Fight to Limit Research of Its DNA, *New York Times*, April 21.

Henderson, L. (2018), The Problem of Induction, *Stanford Encyclopedia of Philosophy* (Spring 2020 Edition), Edward N. Zalta (ed.). Available at: https://plato.stanford.edu/archives/spr2020/entries/induction-problem/.

Hirschman, A. O. (1970), *Exit, Voice and Loyalty: Responses to Decline in Firms, Organizations and State*, Harvard University Press.

Hogle, L. F. (2016), Data-Intensive Resourcing in Healthcare, *BioSocieties*, 11:3, 372–93.

Ippolito, A., Impagliazzo, C., and Zoccoli, P. (2013), Exit, Voice, and Loyalty in the Italian Public Health Service: Macroeconomic and Corporate Implications, *Scientific World Journal*, November 21.

Juengst, E., McGowan, M. L., Fishman, J. R., and Settersten, Jr., R. A. (2016), From "Personalized" to "Precision" Medicine: The Ethical and Social Implications of Rhetorical Reform in Genomic Medicine, *Hastings Center Report*, 46:5, 21–33.

Kelty, C., Panofsky, A., Currie, M. et al. (2015), Seven Dimensions of Contemporary Participation Disentangled, *Journal of the Association for Information Science and Technology*, 66:3, 474–88.

Kitcher, P. (1996), *The Lives to Come: The Genetic Revolution and Human Possibilities*, Simon and Schuster.

Manis, M. L. (2018), La Biobanca Genetica di SharDNA Spa acquistata da Tiziana Life Science PLC: Tutte le tappe della vicenda e le questioni giuridiche da risolvere, *nóva Il Sole 24 Ore*, February 23.

McCoy, M. S., Warsh, J., Rand, L., Parker, M., and Sheehan, M. (2019), Patient and Public Involvement: Two Sides of the Same Coin or Different Coins Altogether?, *Bioethics*, 33, 708–15.

Middleton, A., Niemiec, E., Prainsack, B. et al. (2018), "Your DNA, Your Say": Global Survey Gathering Attitudes toward Genomics: Design, Delivery and Methods, *Personalized Medicine*, 15:4, 311–18.

Middleton, A., Milne, R., Thorogood, A. et al. (2019), Attitudes of Publics Who Are Unwilling to Donate DNA Data for Research, *European Journal of Medical Genetics*, 62, 316–23.

Millikan, R. C. (2006), Commentary: The Human Genome: Philosopher's Stone or Magic Wand? *International Journal of Epidemiology*, 35, 578–80.

Modi, N. (2017), Public Genomes, the Future of the NHS? *The Lancet*, 390, 203.

Osservatorio Donazione Farmaci (2018), *Rapporto 2018: Donare per Curare*, available at: www.bancofarmaceutico.org/cm-files/2018/11/13/rapporto-poverta-2018.pdf.

Peterson A., and Lupton D. (1996), *The New Public Health: Health and Self in the Age of Risk*, Sage.

Prainsack, B. (2017), *Personalized Medicine: Empowered Patients in the 21st Century?*, New York University Press.

Prainsack, B. (2019), Logged Out: Ownership, Exclusion and Public Value in the Digital Data and Information Commons, *Big Data and Society*, January–June, 1–15.

Prainsack, B., Reardon, J., Hindmarsh, R., Gottweis, H., Naue U, Lunshof, J. E. (2008) Personal genomes: Misdirected precaution, *Nature*, 456:7218, 34–35.

Pratt, B. (2018), Constructing Citizen Engagement in Health Research Priority-Setting to Attend to Dynamics of Power and Difference, *Developing World Bioethics*, 1–16.

Rhodes, R. (2005), Rethinking Research Ethics, *American Journal of Bioethics*, 5:1, 19–36.

Rhodes, R. (2008), In Defense of the Duty to Participate in Biomedical Research, *American Journal of Bioethics*, 8:10, 37–8.

Rhodes, R. (2017), When Is Participation in Research a Moral Duty? *Journal of Law, Medicine and Ethics*, 45:3, 318–26.

Rose, N. (2013), Personalized Medicine: Promises, Problems and Perils of a New Paradigm for Healthcare, *Procedia: Social and Behavioral Sciences*, 77, 341–52.

Schaefer, G. O., Emanuel, E. J., and Wertheimer A. (2009), The Obligation to Participate in Biomedical Research, *JAMA*, 302:1, 67–72.

Sen, A. K. (1999), Democracy as a Universal Value, *The Journal of Democracy*, 10:3, 3–17.

Skloot, R. (2010), *The Immortal Life of Henrietta Lacks*, Crown.

Stokstad, E. (2019), Genetics Lab Accused of Misusing African DNA, *Science*, 366:6465, 555–556.

Tutton, R. (2014), *Genomics and the Reimaging of Personalized Medicine*, Ashgate.

Tutton, R., and Prainsack, B. (2011), Enterprising or Altruistic Selves? Making Up Research Subjects in Genetic Research, *Sociology of Health and Illness*, 33:7, 1081–95.

Van Hoyweghen, I. (2007), *Risks in the Making: Travels in Life Insurance and Genetics*, Amsterdam University Press.

Wolf, S. M. (2005), Beyond "Genetic Discrimination": Toward the Broader Harm of Geneticism, in S. A. M. McLean (eds) *Genetics and Gene Therapy*, Routledge.

Woodhouse, E., Hess, D., Breyman, S., and Martin, B. (2002), Science Studies and Activism: Possibilities and Problems for Reconstructivist Agendas, *Social Studies of Science*, 32:2, 297–319.

Woolley, J. P., McGowan, M. L., Teare, H. J. A. et al. (2016), Citizen Science or Scientific Citizenship? Disentangling the Uses of Public Engagement Rhetoric in National Research Initiatives, *BMC Medical Ethics*, 17:33.

3

War on Diseases

Patient Organizations' Problematization and Exploration of Market Issues

Vololona Rabeharisoa and Liliana Doganova

Introduction

Why and how do patient organizations engage with market issues? The answer to the "why" question may sound obvious: in certain countries and/or for certain diseases, patients cannot access drugs because of their high prices. This is what economists call "market failures" which, understandably, prompt patient organizations, as well as non-governmental organizations, to engage with market issues. As for the "how" question, patient organizations, or at least some of them, are often portrayed as lobbies, either allying with the pharmaceutical industry to enlist drugs on public budgets, with the risk of being manipulated by "big pharma," or working hand in hand with public health authorities to slow down the escalating profit-making of pharmaceutical companies.

To date, there is not, strictly speaking, a distinctive body of social science literature on the relationship of patient organizations to the drug market. We have identified two analytical approaches that more or less directly contribute reflections on this topic. The first approach examines the relationship between patient organizations, the pharmaceutical industry, and public authorities.[1] This approach considers patient organizations as a third party in the power struggles between the main actors of the drug market.[2] John Abraham and Courtney Davis' research perfectly illustrates this line of analysis. They have repeatedly pointed to the influence of the pharmaceutical industry on the regulation of the drug market. They have also argued that (de)regulation decisions that have been made by regulatory bodies to accelerate the availability of drugs for unmet medical needs, often upon patients' or patient representatives' requests, have favored "big pharma's" commercial interests

Vololona Rabeharisoa and Liliana Doganova, *War on Diseases: Patient Organizations' Problematization and Exploration of Market Issues* In: *Healthcare Activism: Markets, Morals, and the Collective Good.* Edited by: Susi Geiger, Oxford University Press. © Vololona Rabeharisoa and Liliana Doganova 2021. DOI: 10.1093/oso/9780198865223.003.0003

56   WAR ON DISEASES

to the detriment of public health (Abraham and Davis 2013). One may indeed wonder if certain patients' demands are increasing the power of the industry in directions that may threaten public health systems. As Adriana Petryna (2009) convincingly shows in her exploration of the Brazilian context where universal access to healthcare is a constitutional right, certain patients, sometimes explicitly encouraged by pharmaceutical companies, have sued the federal government in order to obtain highly expensive drugs.[3] So, even if patients and their representatives are successful, it is at the cost of being manipulated by the industry,[4] a phenomenon that may perniciously result in public health systems bankruptcy.

The second approach, drawing inspiration from Michel Callon's analysis of markets (Callon 1998, 2007), has examined patient organizations as groups that are affected by the framing/overflowing of the market, and therefore start to be concerned with it (Callon and Rabeharisoa 2008). Indeed, drug markets can be analyzed as "concerned markets" (Geiger et al. 2014), and patient organizations are emerging as key "concerned groups" that are increasingly willing to address market issues. For instance, when certain non-governmental organizations, as well as patient organizations, publicly denounced the high prices of drugs that hinder their accessibility to poor populations, they started to question the intellectual property regimes that excessively favor the industry to the detriment of those in need, notably in the Global South, as eloquently shown by the 2013 documentary *Fire in the Blood* on spectacular public demonstrations and opposition of people with HIV/AIDS to big pharma in South Africa. Core to these criticisms is the urgent need for alternative licensing schemes, which would allow certain countries to develop their own medications at a lower cost, and/or for adjusted prices that would be affordable for low-income populations. Scholars have studied multiple initiatives from civil society organizations (Cassier and Corrêa 2010; Krikorian 2017; Geiger and Gross 2018), notably patent pools that aim at fighting the retention of molecules needed in multi-therapies by pharmaceutical companies.

The two analytical approaches to the relationship of patient organizations to the drug market that we have identified differ in their understanding of the market. The first approach considers the market as the exclusive playground of the pharmaceutical industry, which is in a unique position to negotiate with public authorities. In this configuration, patient organizations cannot but enter power struggles, and have very little room for maneuver for bringing in substantial changes to the functioning of the market. The second approach considers that the very framing of the market at certain moments and at certain locations provokes its own overflowing at other moments and other locations. Those affected by these dynamics may give shape to their concerns, which the previous framing of the market is unable to absorb, and contemplate a new framing, at least temporarily. This is what certain patient organizations have achieved on the issue of intellectual property regimes. This second approach does not imply a balanced power relationship between patient organizations and the pharmaceutical industry, nor does it suggest that new framings will install themselves smoothly and successfully. What it does highlight is how certain patient organizations come to pay attention to market devices and strive to invent new ones.

Though very different in their intellectual take on the relationship of patient organizations to the drug market, the previous analytical approaches conceive this relationship in terms of patient organizations reacting to the drug market from the outside. They share an understanding of patient organizations as external to the market. Whether they get carried out by market forces beyond their control, embodied by pharmaceutical companies, or concerned by the overflowing of the market, epitomized by the high prices of drugs, patient organizations are envisaged as non-market actors whose engagement with market issues remains sporadic and is driven by exogeneous forces rather than being spontaneously initiated. In this chapter, we argue that this understanding of patient organizations' relation to the drug market proves inaccurate when one considers the case of patient organizations concerned with rare diseases which, from the outset, have been involved in the orphan drug market. More generally, we argue that this understanding does not account (1) for the epistemic role that patient organizations have gradually endorsed throughout their development, and (2) for a range of recent initiatives that extend their epistemic role into the domain of markets. In this chapter, we address these two issues in turn, with the aim of sketching a third approach that analyzes patient organizations as market actors engaged in the construction of markets and in the production of knowledge about markets.

In order to develop our argument, we draw on the literature on patient organizations and on empirical material (documents, ethnographic observations, and interviews) that we have collected on three rare disease patient organizations in France and the United Kingdom (UK), namely:

(1) AFM-Téléthon (French Association against Myopathies), a major player in the area of rare diseases at national and European levels. AFM-Téléthon is the promotor of a few dozens of clinical trials and is involved in negotiations with the French national authorities on issues of accessibility of orphan drugs.

58 WAR ON DISEASES

(2) AKU Society UK, a British charity which partners with a biotech company specializing in orphan drugs for repurposing a molecule against alkaptonuria, an ultra-rare metabolic disease of genetic origin.
(3) EURORDIS (European Organization on Rare Diseases), the umbrella organization of national groups of patients and families concerned with rare diseases in Europe. EURORDIS played a decisive role in the promulgation of the 1999 European Directive on Orphan Medicinal Products. Also, it created EURORDIS Round Table of Companies (ERTC) in 2005; twice a year, ERTC puts together meetings with European and national stakeholders in the area of rare diseases to reflect on the dynamics of research and development (R&D) and the orphan drug market.

In order to better understand why and how rare disease patient organizations intervene in the fabrics of knowledge on economic entities, Section 1 reverts to the epistemic role that patient organizations have forged in Western Europe and North America over the last decades. Based on a synthetic review of the literature on patient activism, we shed light on a significant turn in their epistemic role, when certain patient organizations embraced a new mission that we call "war on diseases" in the 1980s–1990s. We show that in contrast to their traditional missions of mutual support and advocacy for patients' rights, war on diseases leads patient organizations to involve themselves in activities that were long the preserve of specialists, namely biomedical research and therapeutic development. We also show that their engagement takes on a particular form that we call "evidence-based activism" (Rabeharisoa et al. 2014), i.e. the production of knowledge drawn on patients' experience and the confrontation of this experiential knowledge to scientific and medical knowledge with an aim to reform the content and the conduct of R&D on their diseases and give shape to health issues they deem important to address at an individual and a collective level.

Section 2 examines a few recent initiatives that extend patient organizations' evidence-based activism into the domain of markets. We show how the involvement of rare disease patient organizations in therapeutic development has confronted them with market issues, in particular the problems of intellectual property, pricing, and cost evaluation. We discuss in further detail the epistemic work undertaken by the three rare disease patient organizations that we studied on economic entities such as costs and prices. In parallel to conducting clinical trials for repurposing a drug called nitisinone against alkaptonuria, AKU Society UK has engaged in an exploration of the costs of the disease as part of the creation of a referral center where nitisinone is provided off-label to patients. EURORDIS has commissioned a study on the determinants of drug prices in the European Union and regularly puts the issue of orphan drug prices on the agenda of ERTC. AFM-Téléthon has proposed the establishment of an economic observatory of orphan drugs and has put forward the concept of a "fair and controlled price" aiming to reform the mode of calculation of drug prices. We use these three initiatives to show that rare disease patient organizations have extended their evidence-based activism by engaging with economic entities not as a reaction against market forces, but as a series of situated responses to difficulties in the access to medicines in a market that they have actively contributed to create. In line with the epistemic role that they have endorsed throughout their development, the engagement of patient organizations with market issues is deeply intertwined with the production of knowledge about the determinants of prices, the value of drugs, and the definition of diseases alike.

1. The Dynamics of Patient Organizations and Their Epistemic Role

In order to situate rare disease patient organizations' involvement in the fabrics of knowledge on economic entities, it is worth looking at why and how patient organizations have come to endorse an epistemic role, and how this role has evolved over the last decades. This implies a brief incursion into the dynamics of patient organizations. Though there is an abundant literature on patient organizations, there exists no extensive study of their history and their transformation over time. This is probably due to the diversity of patient organizations in terms of their membership, modes of organizing and functioning, causes they defend, and their public positioning vis-à-vis different actors in the domain of health and medicine, as much as the diversity of analytical approaches to patient activism.

Our interest is in the reasons why some patient organizations, whose members do not necessarily possess scientific credentials, have made the decision to intervene in biomedical research, therapeutic development, and the drug market, and how they have contributed to debates and initiatives on topics that have long been the preserve of specialists. This is why we focus our attention on patient organizations that present two characteristics:

(1) These are groups of people directly concerned with a disease, a disability, or a health issue, who gather on a voluntary basis and organize around shared goals. Some of these people may be medical doctors or health professionals, but the important thing is that they belong to these groups either as patients themselves or as patients' relatives and friends.

(2) Within these patient organizations, the decision power on their missions and actions lies in the hands of concerned people, though these organizations may have close relations with specialists, or even in-house scientific committees.

Our definition of patient organizations does not aim to cover all kinds of patient and health activist groups. In light of our research questions, our interest is in organized groups of patients which are patient-led.

When looking at the literature, we can trace back patient organizations' interest in knowledge since their inception in the 1940s–1950s in Western Europe and North America. This manifested in their claiming the importance of what Thomasina Borkman called "experiential knowledge" (Borkman 1976) and in their positioning as epistemic actors, either acting as auxiliaries to medical professionals, or opposing credentialed experts. The 1980s–1990s witnessed a shift in patient organizations' epistemic role when some, including rare disease patient organizations, started to engage in a war on diseases for pragmatic reasons that we illustrate below. Their worry about therapeutic development and their economic impediments is part and parcel of this mission that changes the role they give to experiential knowledge. In particular, they forge a new form of patient activism that we call "evidence-based activism" (Rabeharisoa et al. 2014), which consists in drawing upon experiential knowledge and confronting it to scientific knowledge with an aim to give shape to problems that patients deem crucial to address. It is these few historical landmarks that we would like to sketch out in this section.

1.1 The Rise of Experiential Knowledge in Early Groups of Patients and Disabled People

In the 1940s–1950s, some patients suffering from chronic illnesses formed groups to share their experiences on what it is to live with their diseases. Though chronic illnesses like diabetes or multiple sclerosis benefited from some medical care, at least in Western Europe and North America, patients felt that the biographical disruption (Bury 1982) that their diseases provoked was often overlooked by medical practitioners. Depression, job loss, divorce, and withdrawal from social life featured high on the list of problems they encountered. The groups they formed were places for mutual recognition and capacity building for coping with the diseases and their consequences.

The mode of collective action of these very first patient organizations is similar to the one developed by the self-help/mutual aid movement. It is said that Alcoholics Anonymous was the founding father of this movement in the mid-1930s in the United States (USA). Though Alcoholics Anonymous was not a patient organization strictly speaking, exchanges of experiences between peers made it realize that alcoholism resulted from an addiction to alcohol and not from a lack of volition as some psychiatrists then contended, thus shifting alcoholism from the terrain of deviance to the domain of health. Besides, exchanges of experiences between alcoholics on how to stay sober soon constituted a therapeutic principle, captured by their motto: "You can do it yourself, but you can't do it alone."

In her groundbreaking work on Alcoholics Anonymous and the self-help/ mutual aid movement, Thomasina Borkman (1976) coined the notion of "experiential knowledge" to designate the knowledge that people who share the same condition draw on their experiences and that they collectively elaborate on these in order to better understand their situation and find out solutions to their problems. Experiential knowledge therefore is not only the basis for the social bond between group members; it also denotes the epistemic role played by self-help/mutual aid groups in the understanding of people's conditions.

It is this dual social and epistemic role that groups of patients with chronic illnesses adopted. Experiential knowledge there encompassed the evolution of diseases as well as their "non-technical" dimensions. Interestingly, some medical doctors soon created "therapeutic groups" within hospitals to allow patients to socialize, while preserving professionals' epistemic authority. This translated into a distribution of competences and prerogatives between patients and medical doctors: patients provided mutual emotional and social support, while medical doctors focused on the "technical" aspects of the disease. This distribution was far from peaceful though: the literature reports on numerous examples of conflicts between patients and doctors on the respective values of "experiential knowledge" and credentialed medical knowledge.[5]

This short history of groups of patients with chronic illnesses highlights the significant role of experiential knowledge in the early shaping of patient activism. Experiential knowledge has also been put center stage by groups of disabled people which have multiplied from the 1960s onwards, though in a different way compared to self-help/mutual aid groups. Some fight for social recognition and for their rights as full-fledged citizens being guaranteed by public authorities. Drawing on their lived experiences, they consider that disability is not an individual problem but a social problem that institutions are responsible for. This is best illustrated by people in wheelchairs, who publish testimonies to argue that the problem is not they being unable to walk, but the environment not being designed to facilitate their circulation (Zola 1982). From this perspective, they criticize self-help/mutual aid groups for turning onto themselves, and overtly self-describe as activist groups engaged in power struggles with institutions with an aim at putting their problem on the political agenda.

Other groups of disabled people take on a completely different stance by staging their experience at the core of their identity claim. Deaf communities, studied by Stuart Blume (2010), offer a radical illustration. Stuart Blume shows that deaf people do not consider deafness as a disability, but rather as their very being. They fight for the recognition and perpetuation of their being, rejecting corrective solutions like cochlear implantation. This emancipation vis-à-vis the medical milieu does not equate to an anti-science movement though. Indeed, deaf communities ally with socio-linguistics that demonstrates that sign language is a genuine language and a non-negotiable component of deaf identity and culture.

Groups of disabled people share many features with new social movement organizations, whose origin dated back to the civil rights movements, feminist movements, and gay and lesbian movements in the 1960s–1970s in the USA. Studies on new social movements (Melucci 1980; Touraine 1982) highlight their constituency-based claim: they fight for the recognition of certain categories of the population, which consider that they suffer from stigmatization and exclusion, and ask for socio-political reforms dedicated to their specific conditions. Moreover, certain new social movement organizations of gay and lesbian people combat the understanding of homosexuality either as a disease or as a deviant behavior. They consider that their experience is *the* relevant form of knowledge on their condition, and therefore, that every single action undertaken on their behalf must account for who they are and their views on what they deem legitimate to be done. This dual epistemic and identity claim translates into the motto of these new social movement organizations: "Nothing on us without us."

Beyond groups of disabled people, many patient organizations have also appropriated this motto, so much so that many scholars consider patient organizations as new social movement organizations, which promote a vibrant civil society. And indeed, HIV/AIDS groups of activists (Epstein 1996), the disability rights movement (Winter 2003), and breast cancer groups of activists (Klawiter 2008) stem from new social movements and borrow from their cultures of action.

This picture of new social movements points to the "empowerment" of patient organizations, a complex notion that denotes their self-description as full-fledged actors, able to oppose credentialed experts and policy makers, as much as the contentious legitimacy of their power. This shows in the names of certain groups like ACT UP (AIDS Coalition to Unleash Power). Of note, experiential knowledge here is no longer a means for doing what medical doctors do not do, namely social and emotional support, but a vehicle for empowerment, and in some cases, for emancipation vis-à-vis institutions.

1.2 The Mobilization of Experiential Knowledge in the War on Diseases and the Emergence of "Evidence-Based Activism"

The epistemic role of patient organizations significantly changed in the 1980s–1990s, when some started to engage in what we call a war on diseases. War on diseases is not a new social movement *per se*, and patient organizations which engage in such a war do not necessarily position themselves as activist groups. Rather, war on diseases is a mission that certain patient organizations embrace for very pragmatic reasons. These organizations are indeed concerned with "illnesses they have to fight to get," as Joseph Dumit puts it (Dumit 2006). These are conditions that have either been ignored for political reasons like Gulf War Syndrome at its beginning (Swoboda 2006), conditions on which there was no robust body of knowledge like rare diseases (Rabeharisoa and Callon 2004), emergent conditions like environmental diseases whose etiology is contested (Brown et al. 2006), or unsettled conditions like Attention Deficit Hyperactivity Disorder on which specialists continue to oppose each other in certain countries (Bergey et al. 2018), to cite but a few examples. In these situations, patient organizations are no longer content to provide mutual support or to advocate for patients' rights, interests, and identities; they now designate the disease itself as the object of their mobilization. To achieve their objective, they enter the realm of scientific research in order to enroll specialists in their war on diseases. This is a spectacular watershed in the dynamics of

64 WAR ON DISEASES

patient activism: indeed, these patient organizations get actively involved in domains that have long been the preserve of credentialed experts.

What exactly do they do to get specialists interested in their diseases? Patient organizations collect and format patients' experiential knowledge in order to explore their problems and then confront this experiential knowledge to scientific knowledge in order to identify "zones of undone science" (Frickel et al. 2010) that they feel important to investigate in order to account for patients' problems. This form of activism, which we call "evidence-based activism" (Rabeharisoa et al. 2014), brings in dramatic changes to the distribution of competences and prerogatives between patients and specialists. Indeed, patient organizations are no longer content to act as auxiliaries of medical doctors like self-help/mutual aid groups do, nor do they simply oppose specialists like new social movement organizations do. They rather introduce patients' experiential knowledge and perspectives to specialists, with an aim to transform the very content and conduct of scientific research to the benefit of patients.

Rare disease patient organizations, which are the focus of this chapter, offer a particularly telling example of what evidence-based activism is about. Here, AFM-Téléthon, whose history we studied, stands as a *cas d'école* (Rabeharisoa and Callon 1999). The AFM was created in 1958 by a few parents of children with Duchenne muscular dystrophy, a devastating disease with no treatment. Members of the AFM started to read the scientific literature and to visit hospitals, and became what Steven Epstein (1995) calls "lay experts." The AFM realized that scientific knowledge on myopathies was almost inexistent in France and that very few clinicians knew about these diseases. Because parents refused to give up in the face of this situation, the AFM had no alternative other than producing itself the first corpus of knowledge on myopathies. The AFM collected testimonies from parents, made films, conducted surveys to produce the first clinical descriptions of myopathies, and thus became "experts of experience." They assembled all those facts and presented them to clinicians and researchers. By effecting a confrontation between families' experiential knowledge with the scarce medical and scientific knowledge available at that time, the AFM elicited some interest in the medical and scientific milieu, raised new research questions on which it launched research projects, and later on funded large research programs, thanks to the money it collected through its fundraiser called Téléthon. In doing so, the AFM eventually brought about paradigmatic changes in the understanding of myopathies. For example, a group of parents of children suffering from spinal muscular atrophy were used to exchange their experiences and noticed that the body temperature of their children was lower than normal (36.5°C on average instead of 37.2°C). They alerted clinicians and asked them to figure out the potential causes of this phenomenon. After a series of clinical investigations, it turned out that this low body temperature was related to cardiac problems, though myopathies were not supposed to affect the cardiac muscle. This finding contributed crucial knowledge to a category of diseases called "cardiomyopathies."

Many rare disease patient organizations were confronted with the rareness of knowledge on their conditions, which made it challenging to identify concerned patients. It is this vicious circle of medical and social ignorance that AKU Society UK, a small British charity that we studied, wanted to break down from the start. AKU Society UK was created in 2002 by an adult patient and a clinician at Liverpool Hospital. Its mission is targeted towards war on diseases: to support patients and families concerned with a disease called alkaptonuria, to produce knowledge on its causes and manifestations, and to find a cure. Though alkaptonuria was not unknown, it is an ultra-rare disease on which scientific knowledge was very poor. Alkaptonuria remains silent for many years before visible symptoms manifest; indeed, the only manifestation of the disease is black urine in babies, an extremely frightening phenomenon for young parents but that doctors cannot make sense of because this black urine does not contain blood and babies are usually well. This prompted the chief executive officer of AKU Society UK, the father of two boys with the disease, to put together a website and to publicize alkaptonuria, with an aim to call for testimonies of families who might be concerned with alkaptonuria, collecting their observations on the manifestations of the disease and, above all, counting patients. In 2015, the charity identified sixty-two patients in the UK, a figure that contributed to determine the prevalence of the disease and to complement its description in the same move. This sort of epidemiological study constituted a crucial step on the path to future biomedical research and the search for a treatment, which AKU Society UK engaged with (cf. Section 2). This is also how rare disease patient organizations empower themselves: they are in a position to depict the patient population, a highly valuable asset for researchers, clinicians, and drug manufacturers.

Evidence-based activism does not always provoke substantial disruptions in the understanding of diseases. It does however destabilize existing bodies of scientific knowledge and question the epistemic authority of specialists. Indeed, experiential knowledge here is not restricted to the social and emotional consequences of the disease on concerned people's lives, but encompasses the very description of the disease and of the patient population that

66   WAR ON DISEASES

had long been monopolized by specialists. Experiential knowledge here does not result only from individual introspection into concerned people's subjective experience; it also relies on multiple observations, testimonies, and surveys. Somehow, the elaboration of experiential knowledge is similar yet different from the production of scientific knowledge. This is why evidence-based activism is often fiercely criticized by credentialed experts, who fear that scientific facts run the risk of being contaminated with "anecdotal evidence" (Moore and Stigloe 2009), which will lead to the development of "impure science," to borrow from Steven Epstein (1996).

Throughout our fieldwork on rare disease patient organizations, we have noticed that evidence-based activism and war on diseases co-evolve. Evidence-based activism leads patient organizations to continuously problematize their situation, and to regularly ask themselves about the remaining and/or new obstacles to overcome. As a consequence, war on diseases is a mission whose contours are not defined once and for all. Problems are not given in advance; they are situated, resulting from patient organizations' inquiries into patients' situations and expectations at certain moments and locations.

In our previous study of EURORDIS, which gathers hundreds of national and regional patient organizations (Rabeharisoa and O'Donovan 2014), we have shown that after its contribution to the drafting and the promulgation of the European Directive on Orphan Medicinal Products in 1999, EURORDIS was confronted with the provision of diagnosis and care, which constituted a crucial issue for the inclusion of patients into multi-sited clinical trials and their monitoring in hospitals. EURORDIS realized that in order to combat rare diseases, a global strategy at European level was much needed. In order to promote this idea, EURORDIS conducted a survey on its members called EurordisCare1 in 2007, which has been repeated three times since. The survey collected data on experiences and expectations of patients and their national organizations with regard to diagnosis and access to health services. The results of this survey were reported in a EURORDIS publication entitled *The Voice of 12,000 Patients*. The survey raised a number of criticisms, not only from some experts but also from certain rare disease patient organizations. These criticisms pointed to a series of methodological flaws: some critics noticed that the survey only considered a few dozens of rare diseases, compared to the thousands of rare diseases identified so far; others worried about the bias in the constitution of the sample, for the survey only addressed patients who were members of rare disease patient organizations; still others regretted that some data were provided by professionals, and therefore did not necessarily reflect patients' views.

These were serious criticisms of the representativeness of the study that EURORDIS could not simply put aside. EURORDIS actually recognized the methodological limitations of its survey. However, it defended its objective, which was to collect individual patients' experiences, turn them into matter of fact, confront them to data from different institutions, and eventually identify discrepancies between national health systems, which EURORIDS considered a dramatic bottleneck in the war on rare diseases in Europe. As one staff member of EURORDIS we interviewed explained: "What we're doing is evidence-based advocacy. Our objective is to produce evidence drawing on our members' experiences and expectations, and to mobilize European health authorities on the problems that our evidence gives shape to." Interestingly, European authorities conferred epistemic capacity and representational legitimacy to EURORDIS. As Robert Madelin, the then director general of DG SANCO, stated: "The information provided by EurordisCare Survey Programme has been essential to the sound preparation of the recent Commission Communication on a European Action in the Field of Rare Diseases" (EURORDIS n.d., 3).

The case of EURORDIS illuminates two points: (1) experiential knowledge is not exclusively focused on concerned people's lived experience with their diseases; it is also about their experience of the functioning of health services and the organization of care; and (2) evidence-based activism entails multiple data recouping and crossing to give shape to issues that patient organizations deem relevant and legitimate to address at an individual and a collective level.

Evidence-based activism thus signposts a significant transformation in the dynamics of patient organizations. It implies that patient organizations do not only ask for their problems to be put on the political agenda; they also invite themselves into debates and activities that have not been open to public scrutiny beforehand. In these debates and activities, they assert themselves as relevant and legitimate stakeholders, able to give rise to and document issues that specialists are not necessarily aware of or knowledgeable about.

To recap, this section pinned down a few historical landmarks on the dynamics of patient organizations and their epistemic role. Our objective was not to provide a typology of patient organizations and health movements, but to shed light on why and how certain patient organizations get involved in the production of knowledge on their diseases.

All patient organizations want their experiences to be recognized and taken into account in the treatment of their diseases. Groups of people with chronic illnesses brought in their experiences of the social consequences of their diseases that were often overshadowed by medical doctors, and somehow acted as auxiliaries to specialists. Groups of disabled people pointed to the social determinants of disability that ran counter to the individual model of disability, and often opposed institutions whose approach to disability they deemed irrelevant in regard to their experiences. When some patient organizations, notably those concerned with rare diseases, started to engage in war on diseases, they brought in their experiential knowledge as a genuine knowledge on their diseases, and strived for it to be considered as an object of collective inquiry involving researchers and patients all together.

Thus, patient organizations have long played an epistemic role, whose rationale and conduct are contingent on the diseases they are concerned with, as much as to the medical, social, and political problems they feel are urgent to solve at certain moments and in certain contexts in order for their conditions to be treated according to their experiences and expectations. In this broad landscape, evidence-based activism brings in significant changes in the epistemic role of patient organizations. Firstly, experiential knowledge is no longer a simple addendum to credentialed knowledge, nor is it an alternative form of knowledge in opposition to credentialed knowledge. Patient organizations that develop evidence-based activism consider that experiential knowledge and credentialed knowledge both partake in the fabric of knowledge on their diseases. Secondly, experiential knowledge does not exclusively focus on patients' embodied experiences of diseases, but extends to their experiences of the organization of care and the range of medical practices that they encounter when they navigate hospitals and medical research and health institutions. Thirdly, patient organizations who engage with evidence-based activism deploy a vast range of tools for acquiring and producing knowledge on issues that may sound far removed from patients' immediate concerns and yet is crucial to their war on diseases. As illustrated by rare disease patient organizations, which are the focus of this chapter, patient organizations launch epidemiological surveys to identify concerned people, to collect medical descriptions of their diseases, and to take stock of their experiences with diagnosis and care. They sometimes do so with specialists, enrolling them into their investigation. When it comes to therapeutic development and the drug market, rare disease patient organizations even commission studies from professionals on topics that they feel are underdocumented, particularly pricing issues that they confront on the path to a cure. This is what we now turn to.

2. The Epistemic Work Undertaken by Rare Disease Patient Organizations on Economic Entities

War on diseases is a substantive turn in the mission that patient organizations embrace as well as in their epistemic role. Let us recap the main characteristics of this mission:

(1) War on diseases implies that patient organizations are no longer mere social reaffiliation groups for patients seeking mutual support, nor are they mere lobbies advocating for patients' rights, interests, and identities against credentialed experts and policy makers.

(2) War on diseases leads patient organizations to enter the realms of biomedical research and therapeutic development. In these domains, their power lies in patients' experiential knowledge that they confront to credentialed knowledge to document problems they deem important to address in order to better serve patients. It is this form of activism that we call "evidence-based activism."

(3) War on diseases is a mission whose contours are not defined once and for all. This has to do with the fact that "evidence-based activism" leads patient organizations to continuously problematize their situation, and to regularly ask themselves about the remaining and/or new obstacles to overcome. Problems are not defined in advance; they are situated, in the sense that they result from patient organizations' inquiry into patients' situations and expectations at certain moments and locations.

This latter characteristic is particularly significant, insofar as it helps to capture why and how rare disease patient organizations have engaged with market issues. This is what we examine now. We show how the involvement of patient organizations in therapeutic development has brought them face to face with market issues, namely the problems of intellectual property rights, pricing, and cost evaluation. Initiatives aiming at sharing intellectual property rights have been well documented in the literature. We use our empirical fieldwork to shed light on two other economic entities with which patient organizations have engaged: costs and prices.

70 WAR ON DISEASES

2.1 Patient Organizations' Involvement
in Therapeutic Development

So far, we have focused on patient organizations' intervention in biomedical research in their war on diseases. War on diseases, however, has moving targets: it may be biomedical research, medical practices, therapeutic development, or health insurance, all domains where patient organizations may identify obstacles that they deem critical to remove to better fight against the disease and its consequences on patients' lives. This is particularly true for therapeutic development, to which certain patient organizations have committed themselves from the 1990s onwards.

Drugs are peculiar products, for their development is strictly regulated before their marketing. In many countries, this regulation came into force in the second half of the twentieth century, when clinical trials were put under the jurisdiction of regulatory bodies for the governments to increase their control on the pharmaceutical industry. For certain patient organizations, this regulation constitutes a bottleneck on the path to cure when patients are left with no treatments and are actually dying while a drug slowly moves through the regulatory process. This is why some patient organizations target clinical trials.

One of the most telling examples of activists' involvement in clinical trials is ACT UP's "therapeutic activism" studied by Steven Epstein (Epstein 1995). As he recounts in his book (Epstein 1996), ACT UP realized that if HIV-positive people and AIDS patients were to access molecules rapidly, then they should be included in clinical trials as soon as possible. In order to advocate for early access, which ran counter to US Food and Drug Administration (FDA) regulations, the group started to learn about the conduct of clinical research to be able to discuss new modalities of recruitment of patients with credentialed experts. In addition, the group drew on experiential knowledge that some people may be HIV positive for many years before the disease develops and promoted the use of a surrogate endpoint (the number of T4 cells) for evaluating the efficacy of experimental molecules. In doing so, the group argued for a therapeutic strategy targeting not only the clinical manifestations of the disease, but also its biological pathways.

Therapeutic activism on HIV/AIDS stands as a *cas d'école*, insofar as it contributed to the institutionalization of compassionate protocols, helped to translate patients' experience into new criteria for the evaluation of experimental drugs, and reshuffled the power relations between regulatory bodies, patient organizations, and the pharmaceutical industry. Today, the active role of certain patient organizations in the design and monitoring of clinical trials, and in the process of drug development broadly speaking, is a tangible reality, particularly in the domain of rare diseases.

One example is PXE International, a group of families concerned with a rare genetic disease for which there is no cure, studied by Carlos Novas (2006). The author shows how the group engaged in evidence-based activism of the sort: they collected patients' experience of the disease, confronted it with the scientific and medical literature and involved the members of the group in a large epidemiological study, whose aim was to mobilize researchers around the disease. PXE International also put together a blood and tissue registry that served in the identification of the genetic mutation involved in the disease. More interestingly, the group imposed itself, after tense negotiations, as a co-owner of the patent with Hawaii University in order to have a say in the marketing of future drugs (see also Rapp et al. 2001). This initiative was much publicized as one possible way for patient organizations to secure reasonable prices for drugs. All the investments that PXE International put in different research activities and infrastructures flesh out what Carlos Novas call a "political economy of hope," i.e. the very definition and valuation of the future, not only for patients and their families, but also for researchers and the biotech industry.

AKU Society UK followed a similar path. As we explained above, this organization conducted a sort of epidemiological study that allowed identifying patients and producing knowledge on the prevalence and the characteristics of alkaptonuria. AKU Society UK aimed not only at understanding the disease, but also at finding a cure. Alkaptonuria is a rare genetic disease[6] resulting in the accumulation of homogentisic acid in the body due to the lack of an enzyme that is supposed to break down this acid. This metabolic dysfunctioning causes ochronosis, e.g. the degradation of cartilages that damages joints. In the mid-2000s, AKU Society UK identified a drug called nitisinone licensed for another rare metabolic disease, tyrosinemia type 1, which has similar features to alkaptonuria. Previous clinical research conducted in the USA suggested that nitisinone could reduce the levels of homogentisic acid. Clinical trials were inconclusive, though patients who were put on nitisinone reported that they "felt better."

According to the chief executive officer of AKU Society UK, the American trial failed against the endpoint chosen at the time: an improvement in the functioning of the hip joint. Drawing on patients' experience with alkaptonuria, he hypothesized that this clinical endpoint does not capture the whole story. This prompted AKU Society UK to launch a consortium called

DevelopAKUre, which designed a completely different trial: (1) instead of the clinical endpoint tested in the American trial, they put to the fore a surrogate endpoint, i.e. the reduction of levels of homogentisic acid; (2) they enlarged the sample of subjects included in the trial to patients whose clinical manifestations of the disease varied in nature and in severity; and (3) they put together a protocol for testing the correlation between the dosage of nitisinone, the development stage of the disease, and the time period during which the subject was put on the drug. The clinical trial showed that nitisinone lowered the amount of homogentisic acid by 99 percent, and Sobi, the manufacturer of nitisinone, has applied for a license for its use in alkaptonuria. At the time of writing, the decision of the European Medicines Agency is pending.

These examples show that drug development is no longer a *terra incognita* for rare disease patient organizations. There are today emerging configurations of actors and values that question the power that regulation has historically conferred to the industry on drug development. We should avoid a too-rosy picture though: not all patient organizations have acquired the capacity to navigate regulatory and industrial affairs. As the previous examples suggest, patient organizations have to familiarize with clinical trial protocols, learn about the endpoints for evaluating the efficacy of experimental drugs, launch epidemiological surveys, design and monitor biological registries and data, and immerse themselves into the business technicalities, all of which are topics that may sound alien to the immediate concerns of patients and their relatives. This does not mean that experiential knowledge does not matter anymore. It rather implies that experiential knowledge is no longer restricted to patients' narratives resulting from their introspection into their subjective experience of the disease; it extends to patient organizations' knowledge that they accumulate by conducting their own observations and inquiries into problems that patients are facing in their daily lives, like the absence of adequate treatment for instance. This is how patient organizations' epistemic role has extended into the process of therapeutic development and, as we show now, stretched to issues related to access to medicines in the market for orphan drugs.

2.2 Recalculating Costs, Redefining Diseases

Setting up and conducting clinical trials, then applying for market authorization, is a very lengthy process. The time that it requires stands in sharp contrast with the urgency of patients' medical needs. Therefore, in parallel to the clinical trials conducted by DevelopAKUre, AKU Society UK took the initiative to set up a referral center where nitisinone is provided off-label to patients suffering from alkaptonuria: the Robert Gregory National Alkaptonuria Center, named after the patient who co-founded the charity and located in Liverpool Hospital. In UK "off-label law," a referral center for an unmet medical need can be created as a national health special service. AKU Society UK applied to the National Health Service (NHS) in 2011. Core to AKU Society UK's application was a demand for implementing clinical guidelines that included the provision of nitisinone off-label, monitoring patients, and collecting "real-life" data on the history of the disease under treatment (nitisinone along with pain killers, surgeries, social and psychological support, etc.), including patients' reported outcomes.

The provision of nitisinone off-label was seen both as a temporary answer to a still unmet medical need, and as an opportunity to conduct a longitudinal observation study of patients. The object of this study was not only the clinical manifestation of the disease, but also the economic costs that it entailed. Indeed, the calculation of the costs of the disease was a crucial component of the application to the NHS. In order to justify the creation of a referral center for alkaptonuria, AKU Society UK had to prove that alkaptonuria was worth fighting and that the provision of nitisinone was an economically efficient instrument for that. This led the charity into an exploration of the costs of the disease and confronted it with the problem of cost evaluation. Interestingly, recalculating the costs of the disease entailed redefining what the disease does to patients and to health systems more broadly.

To apply to the NHS Specialized Services, AKU Society UK had to fill in a document that required a series of points to be addressed, among which were: average cost per patient; affordability (including financial details of the current and the proposed provision); value for money compared to alternatives (cost per quality-adjusted life year (QALY) and cost per life year gained); and economic efficiency of provision (demonstrating that the proposed provision would be delivered in the most cost-efficient way). The guidelines indicated that applicants should demonstrate the "net cost" of the service to commissioners, existing "income streams" and "savings," and "the total annual cost burden to society that could be avoided" by providing the proposed service. AKU Society UK was thus faced with the requirement to produce a sophisticated cost-benefit analysis of the provision of nitisinone to patients suffering from alkaptonuria. In the absence of any standard data that could support such a calculation, the patient organization had to perform an inquiry quite similar to the one it had performed a few years earlier on the disease itself—but this time the inquiry was on the costs of the disease.

74 WAR ON DISEASES

AKU Society UK's calculation was based on "real-life data," stemming from two sources: (1) interviews with non-patient members of the charity, "to gain an understanding of the disease and potential costs that the NHS is incurring related to alkaptonuria patients"; and (2) interviews with five patients (that is, about 10 percent of the total number of patients that AKU Society UK had identified), "tracking all health care events that could trigger a cost." The calculation was made by an AKU Society UK volunteer who happened to be a chartered accountant and senior analyst in a large consulting company. It identified and provided a measure for the manifold costs of alkaptonuria, notably the costs of multiple surgeries that patients had undergone, "intangible" costs due to inaccurate diagnosis and inappropriate care, and "indirect" costs related to lost wages and production. The study concluded that a "conservative approximation" of the total costs of alkaptonuria in the UK, including indirect costs, ranges from £1.4 million to 2.0 million per year.[7]

AKU Society UK's calculation of the indirect costs of alkaptonuria challenged the established framing of cost in economic evaluation procedures in the UK. The key metric there is the cost per QALY. QALY is evaluated on the basis of the clinical efficacy of the drug, and on the provision that NICE[8] considers legitimate for patients with the targeted disease. NICE then goes on to calculate the cost per QALY, i.e. the price that the Department of Health will be paying for achieving the QALY. Of note, the UK health system is based on an agreement between the Department of Health and the industry: the industry is free to determine the price it proposes for a drug, on the condition that its return on investment is below a certain threshold. This macro-economic rationale[9] results in a cost per QALY of £20,000 to £30,000 as a reasonable ratio for the Department of Health. Assessed against such metrics, the performance of orphan drugs is poor. Due to the low number of rare disease patients and the difficulty of generating clinical evidence, the cost per QALY of orphan drugs ranges between £300,000 and £400,000, which should lead policy makers to restrict access through the NHS (Tordrup et al. 2014).

AKU Society UK argued that the cost per QALY is not relevant for orphan drugs because of the incommensurable burdens of rare diseases, even though they affect limited proportions of the population.[10] NICE itself seems to acknowledge this problem: in a report on "social value judgments" (NICE 2008), which describes the principles to be followed when deciding on the efficiency (namely, cost-effectiveness) of drugs, NICE restated cost-utility analysis as a key tool for decision making, but added that: "Decisions about whether to recommend interventions should not be based on evidence of their relative costs and benefits alone. NICE must consider other factors when developing its guidance, including the need to distribute health resources in the fairest way within society as a whole."

Interestingly, AKU Society UK's claim is not only about considering "other factors" than costs and benefits. It is about recalculating costs. Initiatives such as this do not call for opting out of economic evaluation, but for reframing the terms of the calculation by redefining the types of entities that are to be taken into account and the relationships between them. The problem of "intangible" and "indirect" costs is crucial in this respect. Measuring these costs entails redefining who is concerned by the disease and in which ways. It also entails producing new types of data stemming from the "real life" of patients. Recalculating the costs of the disease thus becomes an opportunity for redefining what the disease is, and what role patients are to play in the war against it.

2.3 Observing and Reforming Prices

Clinical trials are not only lengthy, but also very expensive. The case of nitisinone is peculiar insofar as it is about repurposing: proving that a drug that already exists can be used for a new indication. Many drugs for rare diseases are highly innovative products that require long years of R&D and, often, complex manufacturing processes. Therefore, even when they have participated in the first steps of R&D, patient organizations generally have to delegate the next steps to other actors, typically biotechnology start-ups and/or pharmaceutical companies. In doing so, they lose control over the resulting drug and, importantly, over its price.

The experience of the AFM with a drug called Zolgensma perfectly illustrates this problem. Approved by the FDA in May 2019, Zolgensma became famous for being the world's most expensive drug. Zolgensma is a gene therapy for infants suffering from spinal muscular atrophy, a rare disease that affects about one in every 10,000 newborns and causes paralysis, breathing difficulty, and, often, death before the age of two. The price that its manufacturer, Novartis, obtained for this one-time treatment was US$2.1 million. Novartis integrated this drug in its portfolio following the acquisition of a biotech start-up called AveXis, which itself had acquired a license for the patent jointly held by the Centre national de la recherche scientifique, the French national research organization, and Généthon, a research laboratory dedicated to the design and development of gene therapies for rare diseases, which was created by the AFM.

76   WAR ON DISEASES

The case of Zolgensma stands out for the price reached by this drug, described by many as the highest price ever reached by a drug. However, it is not an isolated case. Zolgensma came as an alternative to another treatment, named Spinraza, for which Biogen claimed a price of US$750,000 in the first year and US$375,000 in the following years—a claim to which the AFM reacted by observing that "Beyond being the first drug for spinal muscular atrophy, Spinraza would also be the most expensive drug in history."[11] Similarly, a couple of years ago, Cerezyme®, a drug developed by the biotech firm Genzyme for Gaucher disease, was described as one of the most expensive molecules ever developed: indeed, its provision was up to US$400,000 per patient per year, depending on the age of the patient (Côté and Keating 2012). Ironically, some observers (Dolgin 2010) think of orphan drugs as "blockbusters of a new type," which occupy very profitable niche markets due to their high prices. Such prices trigger heated public debates, and raise concerns about the sustainability of the rare diseases business model and the privileges that rare diseases benefit from, to the detriment of other neglected diseases (Saviano et al. 2019). They threaten the accessibility of treatments for those who cannot afford to pay and the sustainability of the healthcare systems.

It should be noted that prices are not a novel problem in the orphan drug market, nor for the patient organizations who played a key role in its creation. The orphan drug market was literally invented from scratch, after legislative measures (the 1983 Orphan Drug Act in the USA; the 1999 Directive on Orphan Medicinal Products in Europe) that aimed at correcting a series of effects of the regulation of drug development. Many scholars have reported on this story (Crompton 2007; Novas 2009; Huyard 2011/12; Rabeharisoa and Doganova 2016; Mikami 2017), highlighting the role of coalitions of actors (medical doctors, pharmaceutical companies, patient organizations, policy makers) that vary across national contexts, who worried about the "drug lag" that the regulation might induce, the exclusion of drugs targeting vulnerable populations (notably children), as well as of "non-profitable" drugs. As Koichi Mikami (2017) rightly points out, "orphaned" drugs have denoted a variety of problems that, according to some actors, have been provoked by the regulatory framing of drug development. That "orphaned" drugs turned into "orphan" drugs (i.e. drugs for rare diseases), and came to epitomize the problem of economically non-viable drugs, was very much the result of historical contingencies, mainly the individual, and later on the collective mobilization of patients and families affected by rare diseases.

Economic incentives and scientific assistance that orphan drug regulations offered were meant to alleviate the unattractiveness of rare diseases for pharmaceutical companies, which reason in terms of metrics such as market size. Their effects manifest in the number of drugs for rare diseases, which has steadily grown over the last decades. In 2015, the FDA approved twenty-one new orphan drugs, that is, nearly half of all new drugs approved for the year, and more than half of all the orphan drugs approved before the Orphan Drug Act was passed. High prices are the flip-side of this success story.

While rare disease patient organizations have been actively involved in the creation of the orphan drug market, they have gradually come to realize that price issues can be of paramount significance. Access to medicines is conditioned not only on the existence of these medicines (and hence on the incentives provided to market actors to engage in their development, production, and marketing), but also on their prices, which need to be affordable for public payers. Today rare disease patient organizations worry both about the risk that public authorities refuse to pay the high prices demanded by biotech and pharma companies, and about the potentially damaging effects of the social criticisms against the exceptional status conferred to orphan drugs.

Whether high prices are inherent to the orphan drug market is a question that rare disease patient organizations have started to explore. Orphan drugs are precisely defined by the small number of patients that they will be able to serve; hence, argue pharmaceutical companies, high prices are needed to compensate for low volumes of sales and allow them to recoup the costs of R&D. In response, rare disease patient organizations have started to scrutinize these pricing mechanisms and have conducted surveys on the rationale for the high prices of orphan drugs, in the spirit of evidence-based activism. We present some of the initiatives implemented by the rare disease patient organizations that we studied, aiming to observe prices and to produce knowledge on how high they are and how high they should be.

In 2010, EURORDIS commissioned a consultancy firm to study the correlations between the prices of orphan drugs and a series of variables that are usually put to the fore to justify the high prices of these drugs, such as the prevalence of diseases, the innovative dimension of molecules, and the number and prices of existing alternative treatments.[12] As a matter of fact, correlations turned out to be inconclusive. Moreover, the study reported on enormous discrepancies of prices across European Union member states due to national specificities of health technology assessment procedures.

In a similar vein, the AFM demanded the creation of an economic observatory of orphan drugs (Observatoire économique du medicament orphelin) within the second French national plan on rare diseases 2011–16. The initiative was ambitious: to collect data on the contributing factors to the cost of treatments, to promote studies on the evaluation of the socio-economic impact of diseases, and to set up a database on the prices of drugs. The objective was to foster reflection and provide sound evidence on the calculation of cost-benefit ratios and prices of drugs, as well as to set up a surveillance tool of the economic rationale of orphan drug development. The French public authorities eventually put the initiative aside, arguing that it did not fit with the roadmap of the French national plan on rare diseases, mostly devoted to facilitating diagnosis, care, and clinical research.

Although it failed, at least temporarily, the initiative paved the way to debates on pricing mechanisms and on the sustainability of the economic model of orphan drug development.[13] Patient organizations play a major role in these debates: they contribute to problematizing the definition of the "price" of drugs, in particular the "value" of drugs for patients and society at large. For example, the AFM has put forward the concept of "fair and controlled price," arguing that the classic business model of pharmaceutical development is not compatible with rare diseases.[14] The prices of orphan drugs, explained to us a representative of the AFM during an interview, should be "fair." He argued that there is no point in containing the budgetary impact of orphan drugs, if only because rare disease patients have long been forgotten and deserve collective investment. However, he warned the industry and public authorities alike that prices should also be put under control. He particularly criticized the opportunistic behavior of certain companies, which game the orphan drug regulation with what he called "salami slicing," i.e. the splitting of one disease into multiple rare conditions for ripping the benefits of orphan designations offered by regulatory bodies. At the time of writing, the AFM is refining its concept of "fair and controlled price" and is notably contemplating the costs of drug development and manufacturing as a potentially more accurate basis for determining the prices of drugs than the "value" that they bring to patients and society.

The concept of "fair and controlled price" nicely captures the aim of initiatives that focus on observing and reforming prices. They redefine the problem of the high prices in the market of orphan drugs by drawing attention to the difficulty of assessing and explaining the level of prices. In this perspective, whether a price is high, and whether it should be so, becomes a matter of empirical investigation and collective deliberation. In other words, observing prices is both an epistemic and a political endeavor, driven by the search for the elusive fair price on the calculation of which agreement can be achieved.

To recap, this section looked at how patient organizations come to engage with market issues as part of their war on diseases. The quest for cure prompts certain patient organizations to involve themselves in therapeutic development, notably in clinical trials for accelerating the availability of treatments for unmet medical needs. They are not mere providers of subjects to be included in clinical trials though; they also intervene in their design and the definition of endpoints in line with patients' experiences of the disease, particularly when endpoints are mired in uncertainties as is the case with many rare diseases.

The availability of drugs is just half the equation; their accessibility is still another concern, especially when the high prices of drugs threaten access for all. This is where patient organizations find themselves faced with market issues. Rare disease patient organizations offer interesting insights into evidence-based activism on these issues. Our empirical fieldwork on AKU Society UK, EURORDIS, and AFM-Téléthon shows how they investigate economic entities such as the costs of the disease, the rationale for the medico-economic evaluation of new treatments, and the prices and pricing mechanism of drugs. In doing so, they aim to renew the assessment of the burden of the disease for the health systems by introducing the costs of the disease for patients and families and redefining what the disease is all about for them (AKU Society UK); they question the ready-made reasoning on the determinants of the prices of drugs that are put to the fore to justify their high amounts to the detriment of patients and public payers in many European countries (EURORDIS); they forge new concepts on what prices should be, both from a technical and from a moral point of view (AFM-Téléthon). They thus extend their evidence-based activism from within the orphan drug market, and raise issues that concern both individual patients and health systems.

Conclusion

In this chapter, we have addressed the question of why and how patient organizations engage with market issues. Classic approaches to this question consider patient organizations as aliens to the drug market, only reacting from the outside to its undesirable effects on patients, such as the lack of accessibility of certain drugs because of their high prices. Our focus on rare disease patient organizations has helped us to explore an alternative approach to the relationship between patient organizations and the drug market. Indeed, rare disease patient organizations have been full-fledged actors of the market from the outset, when they contributed to the promulgation of legislations on orphan medicinal products as part of the war on diseases they have engaged

80   WAR ON DISEASES

in for decades. For this reason, they are interesting loci for examining patient activism from within the market.

Today, the high prices of drugs are a major concern for patient organizations and for health systems alike. Rare disease patient organizations are even more preoccupied by the problem of drug prices because some voices start to call for a radical revision of orphan drug legislations that constitute the pillar of the orphan drug market and that they have proactively promoted and continue to defend. In this situation, some rare disease patient organizations have started to scrutinize the very pricing mechanisms as well as the cost-effectiveness calculations of orphan drugs. It is this epistemic work undertaken by rare disease patient organizations on a series of economic entities that this chapter has documented and analyzed. Our inquiry has been on patient organizations' own inquiries into knowledge about economic entities. This approach has helped us to enrich the corpus of research works on what we call evidence-based activism, that is the involvement of patient organizations into the production, discussion, and circulation of different corpus of knowledge on issues they deem crucial to tackle for better serving the patients.

Our perspective has also offered a more nuanced understanding of the relationship of patient organizations with the drug market. The rare disease patient organizations that we studied can hardly be depicted as organizations manipulated by the industry; they are of course aware of the risk of an unfair relationship with biotech companies and pharmaceutical corporations, but they have cooperated with them from the beginning in order to foster therapeutic R&D and to give shape to the orphan drugs market. Neither can rare disease patient organizations be considered as concerned groups reacting from the outside to the overflowing of the orphan drugs market; they are certainly concerned by this overflowing, but they have been part of the framing of this market from the outset. Our approach consists in taking into consideration the reflexive and situated investigation that rare disease patient organizations engage on and from within the orphan drug market, at this particular moment when the dynamics of this market threaten their efforts to make it economically viable and socially meaningful.

It is worth saying a final word on the moral positioning of the rare disease patient organizations we investigated. In contrast to lay and expert critics against the commodification of health, these patient organizations do not reject the market as a way to access drugs. Quite the contrary: for them, caring about the market is part and parcel of caring about the patients. Indeed, as some patients' representatives point out, market issues, and particularly the pricing of drugs, are the most sensitive political bastions on the path to cure, for they shed a harsh light on the frictions between individual interests and the common good. Consequently, patient organizations, though adamant that the high prices of drugs should be combatted by all means, move on to a much more fundamental question: what is a "good price," and who should be entitled to determine it? This is why they conduct surveys and strive to bring in data and evidence to document economic issues that are even more contentious than scientific issues. For this reason, exploring their own studies is a means of penetrating into the actual making of economic entities.

Notes

1. Public authorities include regulatory bodies which deliver market approvals to new drugs, and health technology assessment agencies which evaluate their cost-effectiveness.
2. In the United States, we have to add the insurance companies and the health management organizations, which determine the drugs that their individual and corporate clients may access through their insurance policies.
3. Adriana Petryna adds that the picture is worsened by the powerlessness of the Brazilian federal government, which has very few health technology assessment capacities, and therefore, very little room for maneuver for evaluating the efficacy and efficiency of drugs.
4. Some scholars have questioned this "corporate colonization" of patient activism, showing that patient organizations are not condemned to be puppets in the hands of the pharmaceutical industry. In a survey of 112 Irish patient organizations, followed by qualitative research with a few of them, Orla O'Donovan provides evidence on patient organizations either opposing pharmaceutical corporations or engaging a cautious relationship with them, depending on their cultures of action, i.e. their constructions of the health cause around which they are organized, the kind of patienthood they espouse, their ways of taking political action, and their framings of friends and foes (O'Donovan 2007). While she recognizes that some patient organizations may be the instruments of big pharma's expansion, her study opens a breach in the narrative of patient organizations being dominated and manipulated by corporations.
5. In this respect, Francine Lavoie, Thomasina Borkman, and Benjamin Gidron (1994) edited a handbook to help professionals collaborate with self-help/mutual aid groups.
6. The prevalence of alkaptonuria is estimated at one person in 250,000 to one person in 500,000 (see http://www.akusociety.org/what-is-alkaptonuria).
7. These calculations were included in AKU Society UK's application to the Advisory Group for National Specialised Services, June 2011: 18. With courtesy of AKU Society UK.
8. National Institute for Health and Care Excellence. NICE is the UK health technology assessment agency.
9. On QALY and health economics in the UK, see Moreira (2012).

82   WAR ON DISEASES

10. Many rare disease patient organizations put forward this argument, see e.g. Rare Disease UK (2011).
11. AFM-Téléthon, 10 January 2017, "Spinraza: l'AFM-Téléthon se réjouit de cette avancée majeure pour les malades mais demande à Biogen de faire toute la transparence sur le prix revendiqué," https://www.afm-telethon.fr/actualites/spinraza-afm-telethon-se-rejouit-cette-avancee-majeure-pour-malades-mais-demande-biogen. On the influence of social media on the decision making in Ireland's Spinraza reimbursement process, see Moran and Mountford in this volume.
12. The results of the study were presented in the report of EURORDIS Round Table of Companies 13th Meeting, entitled "Patients' Access to Orphan Medical Products, Innovative Pricing Schemes, and National Measures in Global Financial and Economic Crisis Environment" (December 13, 2010). With courtesy of EURORDIS.
13. See for instance RARE 2013, Les Rencontres Eurobiomed des Maladies Rares: L'innovation et les partenariats au service des malades, 3rd edition (Montpellier, November 28–29, 2013), *Medecine/Science* 30: 21–23, April 2014.
14. RARE 2015, Les Rencontres Eurobiomed des Maladies Rares: Les maladies rares: quelles attentes et quels enjeux pour la société?, 4th edition (Montpellier, November 26–27, 2015), *Medecine/Science* 32: 11, April 2016.

References

Abraham, J. and Davis, C. (2013), *Unhealthy Pharmaceutical Regulation. Innovation, Politics and Promissory Science*, Palgrave Macmillan.

Bergey, M. R., Filipe, A. M., Conrad, P., and Singh, I. (2018), *Global Perspectives on ADHD*, Johns Hopkins University Press.

Blume, S. (2010), *The Artificial Ear: Cochlear Implants and the Culture of Deafness*, Rutgers University Press.

Borkman, T. (1976), Experiential Knowledge: A New Concept for the Analysis of Self-Help Groups, *Social Service Review*, 50:3, 445–56.

Brown, P., McCormick, S., Mayer, B. et al. (2006), "A Lab of Our Own": Environmental Causation of Breast Cancer and Challenges to the Dominant Epidemiological Paradigm, *Science, Technology and Human Values*, 31, 499–536.

Bury, M. (1982), Chronic Illness as Biographical Disruption, *Sociology of Health and Illness*, 4:2, 167–82.

Callon, M. (1998), *The Laws of the Markets*, Blackwell.

Callon, M. (2007), An Essay on the Growing Contribution of Economic Markets in the Proliferation of the Social, *Theory, Culture and Society*, 24:7–8, 139–63.

Callon, M., and Rabeharisoa, V. (2008), The Growing Engagement of Emergent Concerned Groups in Political and Economic Life: Lessons from the French Association of Neuromuscular Disease Patients, *Science, Technology and Human Values*, 33:2, 230–61.

Cassier, M., and Corrêa, M. (2010), Brevets de médicament, lutte pour l'accès et intérêt public au Brésil et en Inde, *Innovations*, 2:32, 109–27.

Côté A., and Keating B. (2012), What Is Wrong with Orphan Drug Policies? *Value in Health*, 15, 1185–91.

Crompton, H. (2007), Mode 2 Knowledge Production: Evidence from Orphan Drug Networks, *Science and Public Policy*, 34:3, 199–211.

Dolgin E. (2010), Big Pharma Moves from Blockbusters to Niche Busters, *Nature Medicine*, 16:8, 837.

Dumit, J. (2006), Illnesses You Have to Fight to Get: Facts as Forces in Uncertain, Emergent Illnesses, *Social Science and Medicine*, 62, 577–90.

Epstein, S. (1995), The Construction of Lay Expertise: AIDS Activism and the Forging of Credibility in the Reform of Clinical Trials, *Science, Technology and Human Values*, 20, 408–37.

Epstein, S. (1996), *Impure Science: AIDS, Activism, and the Politics of Knowledge*, University Press of California.

EURORDIS (n.d.), The Voice of 12,000 Patients. Available at: www.eurordis.org/publication/voice-12000-patients.

Frickel, S., Gibbon, S., Howard, J., Kempner, J., Ottinger, G., and Hess, D. J. (2010), Undone Science: Charting Social Movement and Civil Society Challenges to Research Agenda Setting, *Science, Technology, and Human Values*, 35:4, 444–73.

Geiger, S., and Gross, N. (2018), Market Failures and Market Framings: Can a Market Be Transformed from the Inside? *Organization Studies*, 39:10, 1357–76.

Geiger, S., Harrison, D., Kjellberg, H., and Mallard, A. (eds) (2014), *Concerned Markets: Economic Ordering of Multiple Values*, Edward Elgar Publishing.

Huyard, C. (2011/12), Quand la puissance publique fait surgir et équipe une mobilisation protestataire. L'invention des "maladies rares" aux Etats-Unis et en Europe, *Revue française de sciences politiques*, 61, 183–200.

Klawiter, M. (2008), *The Biopolitics of Breast Cancer: Changing Cultures of Disease and Activism*, University of Minnesota Press.

Krikorian, G. P. (2017), From AIDS to Free Trade Agreements: Knowledge Activism in Thailand's Movement for Access to Medicines, *Engaging Science, Technology, and Society*, 3, 154–79.

Lavoie, F., Borkman, T., and Gidron, B. (eds) (1994), *Self-Help and Mutual Aid Groups: International and Multicultural Perspectives*, Haworth Press.

Melucci, A. (1980), The New Social Movements: A Theoretical Approach, *Social Science Information*, 19:2, 199–226.

Mikami, K. (2017), Orphans in the Market: The History of Orphan Drug Policy, *Social History of Medicine*, 32:3, 609–30.

Moore, A., and Stilgoe, J. (2009), Experts and Anecdotes: The Role of "Anecdotal Evidence" in Public Scientific Controversies, *Science, Technology and Human Values*, 34:5, 654–77.

Moreira, T. (2012), *The Transformation of Contemporary Health Care: The Market, the Laboratory, and the Forum*, Routledge.

NICE (2008), Social Value Judgements: Principles for the Development of NICE Guidance (2econd edition). Available at: https://www.nice.org.uk/media/default/about/what-we-do/research-and-development/social-value-judgements-principles-for-the-development-of-nice-guidance.pdf.

Novas, C. (2006), The Political Economy of Hope: Patients' Organizations, Science and Biovalue, *BioSocieties*, 1, 289–305.

Novas, C. (2009), Orphan Drugs, Patient Activism and Contemporary Healthcare, *Quaderni*, 68, 13–23.

O'Donovan, O. (2007), Corporate Colonization of Health Activism? Irish Health Advocacy Organizations' Modes of Engagement with Pharmaceutical Corporations, *International Journal of Health Services*, 37:4, 711–33.

Petryna, A. (2009), *When Experiments Travel: Clinical Trials and the Global Search for Human Subjects*, Princeton University Press.

Rabeharisoa, V., and Callon, M. (1999), *Le Pouvoir des maladies. L'Association Française contre les Myopathies et la Recherche*, Les Presses des Mines.

Rabeharisoa, V., and Callon, M. (2004), Patients and Scientists' French Muscular Dystrophy Research, in S. Jasanoff (ed.) *States of Knowledge: The Co-Production of Science and Social Order*, Routledge, 142–60.

Rabeharisoa, V., and O'Donovan, O. (2014), From Europeanization to European Construction: The Role of European Patients' Organizations in the Shaping of Health-Care Policies, *European Societies*, 16:5, 717–41.

Rabeharisoa, V., and Doganova, L. (2016), Making Rareness Count: Testing and Pricing Orphan Drugs, *i3 Working Papers Series*, 16-CSI-03.

Rabeharisoa, V., Moreira, T., and Akrich, M. (2014), Evidence-Based Activism: Patients', Users' and Activists' Groups in Knowledge Society, *BioSocieties*, 9:2, 111–28.

Rapp, R., Heath, D., and Taussig K.-S. (2001), Genealogical Dis-ease: Where Hereditary Abnormality, Biomedical Explanation, and Family Responsibility Meet, in F. Franklin and S. McKinnon (eds) *Relative Values: Reconfiguring Kinship Studies*, Duke University Press, 384–409.

Saviano, M., Barile, S., Caputo, F., Lettieri, M., and Zanda, S. (2019), From Rare to Neglected Diseases: A Sustainable and Inclusive HealthCare Perspective for Reframing the Orphan Drug Issue, *Sustainability*, 11.

Swoboda, D. A. (2006), The Social Construction of Contested Illness Legitimacy: A Grounded Theory Analysis, *Qualitative Research in Psychology*, 3, 233–51.

Tordrup D., Tzouma V., and Kanavos P. (2014), Orphan Drug Considerations in Health Technology Assessment in Eight European Countries, *Rare Diseases and Orphan Drugs: An International Journal of Public Health*, 1:3, 86–97.

Touraine, A. (ed.) (1982), *Mouvements sociaux d'aujourd''hui. Débats dirigés par Alain Touraine*, Les éditions ouvrières.

Winter, J. A. (2003), The Development of Disability Rights Movement as a Social Solving Problem, *Disability Studies Quarterly*, 23:1, 33–61.

Zola, I. K. (1982), *Missing Pieces: A Chronicle of Living with a Disability*, Temple University Press.

4

"Please Don't Put a Price on Our Lives"

Social Media and the Contestation of Value in Ireland's Pricing of Orphan Drugs

Gillian Moran and Nicola Mountford

Introduction

Social media play an ever increasing role in the organization of collective action where property rights, actors, networks, and governance are enacted and contested by political, cultural, and social institutions (Dacin et al. 1999). Social media's role in building community (Kaplan and Haenlein 2010) and facilitating advocacy (Obar et al. 2012) is well charted, as is the ubiquity of social media in our daily lives (Hewett et al. 2016).

Our goal is to understand how organizations and individuals alter definitions of value within the pharmaceutical market through their actions and interactions on social media. We examine social media influence in two case studies in the context of Irish drug pricing. The drugs in both cases fall into a special category—that of orphan drugs. In the European Union, orphan drugs are classified as those that are designed for the diagnosis, prevention, or treatment of life-threatening conditions that affect no more than five in 10,000 people. Their special status means that those who develop and produce orphan drugs benefit from a wide range of support including public funding for basic science, tax incentives, extended patent protection, and market exclusivity.

In 2013, the Irish government gave full statutory powers to the Health Service Executive (HSE) to make decisions on the reimbursement of medicines through the Health (Pricing and Supply of Medical Goods) Act 2013. The Act specifies the criteria to be applied in assessing the value of all new drugs including the clinical and cost-effectiveness of the product, opportunity costs, and impact on resources available. The HSE is required to take the advice of the National Centre for Pharmacoeconomics (NCPE) in making its decisions. Our first case deals with the provision of the drug Orkambi for cystic fibrosis (CF) patients. Orkambi was approved for access in Ireland

Gillian Moran and Nicola Mountford, *"Please Don't Put a Price on Our Lives": Social Media and the Contestation of Value in Ireland's Pricing of Orphan Drugs* In: *Healthcare Activism: Markets, Morals, and the Collective Good.* Edited by: Susi Geiger, Oxford University Press. © Gillian Moran and Nicola Mountford 2021. DOI: 10.1093/oso/9780198865223.003.0004 following eleven months of public debate and social media campaigning by people living with CF, their loved ones, and their advocates. The second case concerns the provision of the Spinraza drug for patients with spinal muscular atrophy (SMA). Spinraza was also approved for access after "a lengthy campaign by patients and their families."[1] In both cases, the HSE and NCPE had initially refused reimbursement.

In the wake of these and other similar campaigns, Bill 33 of 2018, an amendment to the Health Act (2013), was debated in the Irish parliament (Dáil). The Bill was an attempt to change the existing reimbursement decision-making process for orphan drugs only. It proposed that "guidelines which include a threshold cost-effective incremental ratio or similar assessment, shall not be relevant in the case of Orphan Medicinal Products." In other words, the objective clinical/cost assessment process outlined in the original 2013 Act would not be applied to orphan drugs. This proposal was not universally popular. Indeed, Professor Michael Barry, Director of Ireland's NCPE, has argued that "it will not help a single patient" and will only lead to massive hikes in the cost of medicines: "What it is saying, is the highest cost drugs that we look at every day—that cost more than half-a-million euro per patient per year—we are not allowed to ask about cost-effectiveness?"[2]

We ask what role social media activism played in this new bill that aimed to alter the processes by which value was calculated for this subsection of drugs. The chapter is structured as follows. We first review and synthesize the social media literature, linking it to its use in the contestation of value, particularly in the context of healthcare markets. Second, we describe how we used social media data to build a picture of social media influence on reimbursement decision making within the Irish market for orphan drugs. We focus in particular on the use of social media for information circulation, community building, and mobilization towards action within an online advocacy campaign. Section 3 presents the results of this research in the form of two case studies on the Orkambi and Spinraza campaigns. Drawing on these case studies Section 4 discusses the insights for healthcare market activism arising from our research.

1. The Role of Social Media in Healthcare Market Advocacy

1.1 The Increasing Role of the Market in Healthcare

Marketization often causes fields such as healthcare to seem like markets— subjugating other institutional structures such as state, community, or professions to the market in terms of how value is defined (Thornton 2002). The result is that social relations between doctors and patients may be simplified to that of supplier/consumer (Giroux 2004). The contractual arrangements and monitoring processes that frame the modern healthcare field—such as the reimbursement decision-making process at the heart of our cases—are often shaped by market logics and thus serve to diffuse market principles (Djelic and Sahlin-Andersson 2006). The public sector increasingly commissions while the private sector delivers, resulting in the marketization of healthcare services (Acerete et al. 2012). Acerete et al. offer evidence from Spain where a 2011 report called for management reform in hospitals and a move to a market-based system (Fundación Bamberg 2011) and the United Kingdom where, in 2012, a private healthcare partnership won a £1 billion ten-year deal to run clinical and non-clinical services at Hinchingbrooke Hospital. This reflects an increasingly prevalent "culture of markets" in healthcare where value is perceived through the more efficient allocation of most if not all goods and resources (Djelic 2012).

As Geiger in her introduction to this volume suggests, however, this process is potentially incompatible with civic values and accountability as it places little or no value on democratic ideals such as fairness and justice (Eikenberry and Kluver 2004). Public actors, therefore, continue to bring the state into the market through both legislative and non- legislative methods (Mountford 2019), while other actors including affected patients work to have their voices heard within such "concerned markets" (Geiger et al. 2014). Within healthcare markets the state can play multiple roles—it may act as one large buyer or seller (Ahrne et al. 2015), it can seed and manage relationships (Mountford 2019), and it legislates and makes market rules. This means that, even within a marketized healthcare field, the state remains a target for advocates or activist networks who wish to change the way purchasing decisions are made, challenge the relationships between organizations, or overturn the rules that govern both market and field (Mountford and Geiger 2020). Hoffman (1999) portrayed the field as a center of debate where reconfigurations and reorganizations result from events that trigger new debates or new forms of debate. Patient groups in the United States, for example, advocated for the passage of the American Orphan Drug Act in a bid to encourage the pharmaceutical and biotechnology industry to develop treatments for rare diseases (Novas 2009). Value can become an issue for debate, where new valuation categories go beyond immediate economic valuations to include more complex approaches to valuation that can include emotion, longer-term horizons, or wider impact evaluations (Dubuisson-Quellier 2013). Moreover, social media offer new virtual discursive spaces where texts that shape such new valuation categories can be produced, distributed and consumed (Hajer 1995), and be contested by multiple voices (Hauser 1999).

1.2 Social Media and Healthcare Activism

Social networking sites bring together like-minded individuals, separated by geography or other barriers, to connect and converse over a shared interest or issue (Kaplan and Haenlein 2010). In the healthcare field, patient communities are flourishing on social media (Attai et al. 2015). Virtual patient communities are important sources of emotional support, advice, and camaraderie among those facing comparable illnesses and challenges (Smailhodzic et al. 2016), such that patients may feel "an intrinsic connection toward other members" of the online patient community (Bagozzi and Dholakia 2002, 5). Community members utilize social media as discursive spaces to share latest research and facilitate patient-specific discussions (Dholakia et al. 2004). Social media thus fulfill important identity, community-building, and support functions for patient communities—functions that, as Rabeharisoa and Doganova in their chapter suggest, have always been important to patient organizations and that are now much facilitated through the ubiquity of online tools.

Of late, social media have moved from connecting and exchanging information to becoming central to the instigation and coordination of contemporary advocacy campaigns (Velasquez and LaRose 2015). Advocacy here refers to the "systemic effort by specific actors who aim to further or achieve specific policy goals" by informally influencing public policy (Obar et al. 2012, 4). They facilitate the forming of advocate communities due to their inherent open access, their ability to allow individuals to forge social connections with similar others (Tajfel 1978), and their provision of access to essential resources such as knowledge sharing, advice, and the opinions of experienced others (McAlexander et al. 2002). This empowers users to leverage social media networks to "influence their peers and thus contribute to broader public advocacy efforts that may in fact have real, if indirect, macro-level policy effects" (Penney 2015, 53).

Patient-led advocacy campaigns use social networking sites to present patients' own personalized experiences and struggles to the public, thus putting a human face on a social issue to gain support and solidarity from peers and the wider public. Patient advocates confer both moral authority and public trust on the advocacy cause through the depiction of their ongoing battles with illness (McDonnell 2016). Personalized, emotionally charged health messages propagate quickly online, activating others to get behind an advocacy campaign to help amplify those messages and call for policy change to better the lives of patients (Berger and Milkman 2012; Meng et al. 2018). Online platforms such as Facebook and Twitter facilitate the high-speed diffusion of user-generated information in real time to support such calls for action. This instantaneous communication medium lends a sense of urgency to a campaign, while a community of active members can broadcast and amplify a tidal wave of issue-specific information to attract the attention and influence of multiple public stakeholders (Obar et al. 2012; Poell and van Dijck 2015; Rost et al. 2016).

Social networking site conditions, for instance a dense, well-connected network of people sharing similar interests, provide an incubator for social challenges and online advocacy (Housley et al. 2018). A coordinated campaign that focuses on a specific topic, such as patient welfare, can create a dispro-portionate presentation of that topic in the social media environment (Johnen et al. 2018). This helps to create a narrative for the advocacy campaign through the development of consistent patient-centered messages. When content such as this gains traction and "trends" across social media sites it signals the popularity and importance of the information, which focuses public attention on the campaign's central issue (Meng et al. 2018). Routine social media reactions, such as liking or retweeting content, easily engage people in infor-mation exchange, raising awareness and visibility of an advocacy campaign among previously uninformed peers (Penney 2015; Housley et al. 2018; Moran et al. 2019). In essence, a social media advocacy campaign gently nudges peer connections to advocate for a worthy cause in a participatory, bottom-up approach that garners grassroots social support to subtly shift public opinion (Zuckerman 2014; Penney 2015; Housley et al. 2018).

The relationships between the pharmaceutical industry, state agencies, and patient organizations are key in the framing of the healthcare market (Abraham 2009). Social media have the capacity to transform power rela-tions within the public and civic spheres by bringing in new voices to effect change in regulations or market activities (Soule 2012; Housley et al. 2018), thus "activist organizations are increasingly seeing the value of social media for recruitment, public engagement, and campaign organization" (Murthy 2018, 2). Patients, through activities such as "lobbying, hypermedia cam-paigns and marches," can leverage social media to influence power holders (Acosta 2012, 159; Kraemer et al. 2013). As we will see below, collective action by patient communities can extend to efforts to change field rules as social media provide discursive spaces for patient groups to have their voices included in debating and reframing the meaning of value in the healthcare market.

We argue that these new approaches to, and definitions of, value are developed by community collective action in new social media-based spaces through bringing market-specific issues into the public domain and highlighting competing definitions of value between the patient community and other market actors. A patient community view of value may serve to displace traditional economic valuation in the healthcare market. The social media literature builds a strong case for the role of social media in creating patient communities within healthcare and active communities in markets beyond healthcare. The literature describes how healthcare has become more subject to market culture and how actors can act to shape that market. This chapter seeks to build on both perspectives to focus on the role of social media in patient advocacy campaigns within the healthcare field (Obar et al. 2012; Penney 2015; Housley et al. 2018).

2. Our Research

Case studies have been shown to be particularly suited to how and why questions, to real-life contexts, and to the building of theory (Eisenhardt 1989). Following the case study approach (Yin 2014), we present two cases depicting how the decision-making process for reimbursement approval of orphan drugs in the Irish healthcare market was influenced, and eventually overturned, by a small group of active patients using social media to inform, activate, and mobilize support for their advocacy campaigns. Below is a brief overview of the two cases at the center of our study.

2.1 Orkambi

For all intents and purposes, cystic fibrosis is an Irish disease. We have the highest incidence worldwide. We have some of the most severe CF genotypes...Therefore, we have a duty and responsibility to lead from the front when it comes to CF treatment and care. (Barry Plant, Director of the Adult Cystic Fibrosis Centre at Cork University Hospital, Chairman of Cystic Fibrosis Ireland's Medical and Scientific Committee)[3]

CF is an inherited chronic disease caused by a defective gene that leads to life-threatening lung infections. In 2017, there were 1,237 men, women, and children living with CF in Ireland with a median age of 20.6 years (70,000 worldwide).[4] The outlook for patients suffering from CF has changed dramatically over the past sixty to seventy years. As Cystic Fibrosis Ireland (CFI), states:

> In the 1950s, few children with cystic fibrosis lived to attend primary school. Today, advances in research and medical treatments, including in Ireland, have further enhanced and extended life for children and adults with CF. Many people with the disease in Ireland can now expect to live into their 30s, 40s and beyond.[5]

The number of CF patients in Ireland and across the world is, therefore, forecast to increase as survival rates improve (Burgel et al. 2015).

In 2015, Orkambi, a new drug to treat CF, was brought to market by Vertex Pharmaceuticals and received approval from the FDA. Rather than treat the symptoms of CF, Vertex claims that Orkambi deals with the underlying genetic defect that causes this disease. In Ireland, Orkambi was initially submitted for review to the NCPE on November 26, 2015, and the rapid assessment concluded in December with a recommendation for a full pharmacoeconomic evaluation. This full evaluation commenced on March 11, 2016 and completed on June 1, 2016 with the recommendation that the drug not be reimbursed at the submitted price (€159,000 per patient).

2.2 Spinraza

SMA is a rare disease affecting the motor nerve cells in the spinal cord. It is "a life-threatening and debilitating disease that causes progressive muscle weakness and loss of movement due to muscle wasting," from the same family as motor neuron disease.[6] SMA makes it difficult or impossible to walk, eat, or breathe and affects approximately one in 11,000 babies. About one in every 50 Americans is a genetic carrier. If untreated, one type of SMA (SMA1) can be fatal and is considered the number one genetic cause of death in infants.[7] Most sufferers are confined to a wheelchair and may require mobility/feeding/breathing assistance. In Ireland, twenty-five children and eighteen adults are currently living with SMA.[8]

Spinraza, brought to market by Biogen, is a treatment for SMA, described by the SMA patient community as "the first-ever approved treatment that targets the underlying genetics of SMA."[9] The European Medicines Agency in its approval of the drug therapy referred to studies in early onset SMA patients that have demonstrated its effectiveness in improving movement in babies including head control, rolling, sitting, crawling, standing, and walking. The babies in this study receiving Spinraza also survived longer and deferred needing breathing support until much later.[10]

In Ireland, the NCPE commenced its rapid review process for the Spinraza drug on July 11, 2017. This review completed on August 2, 2017 and recommended a full pharmacoeconomic evaluation. The NCPE completed its full evaluation assessment on December 19, 2017, concluding with the recommendation that Spinraza not be reimbursed at the submitted price (€600,000 for the first year and €380,000 per patient per year thereafter).[11]

2.3 This Study

We focus on the aftermath of the HSE's refusal to reimburse Orkambi and Spinraza. We analyze social media advocacy campaigns led by Irish CF and SMA patients and supporters to challenge these decisions. We focus on Twitter as the dominant social media platform for facilitating advocacy campaigns and shaping public discourse about social issues (Murthy 2018). Certain features of the Twitter ecosystem such as retweets, replies, and hashtags help to connect like-minded individuals, frame a topic by linking conversations together, and depict the temporal sequence of events as they unfold (Housley et al. 2018). Using a Twitter application programming interface, we retrieved and downloaded all tweets sent by the Twitter handles @YesOrkambi and @SMAIrelandCom. These handles represent the patient heart of these advocacy campaigns as they were launched specifically to advocate for the reimbursement of the Orkambi and Spinraza drugs.

In the case of Orkambi, the @YesOrkambi handle launched on June 2, 2016—the day after the HSE's initial refusal decision—with the sole purpose of getting this decision overturned.[12] Led by the mother of a CF patient, the Twitter campaign states: "Orkambi is a breakthrough drug that could change the lives of 600 Irish PWCF [people with CF]. We won't rest until we get access to it—you can't put a price on people's lives."[13] For Spinraza, the @SMAIrelandCom Twitter handle and advocacy campaign took a little longer to begin with, launching on September 12, 2018, nearly nine months after the HSE's decision to refuse reimbursement. It clearly sets out its stall as a campaign to secure HSE funding for SMA-related drugs in Ireland, while its accompanying campaign website reinforces this mandate, stating: "The #SpinrazaNOW campaign is a campaign to ensure that the revolutionary drug Spinraza is available to Irish SMA sufferers through the HSE. This drug is to date the only approved treatment for Spinal Muscular Atrophy and is a lifeline to those suffering from this degenerative disease."[14]

In both cases, we followed the temporal unfolding of these advocacy campaigns on Twitter by analyzing their tweets, including replies and retweets, from initial launch until the drug reimbursement was eventually approved by the HSE. In total, we analyzed 1,012 tweets by @YesOrkambi and 247 tweets by @SMAIrelandCom. In coding using NVivo software, we followed Krippendorff's (2013) guidelines for quantitative content analysis manifest in the objective observation of deductive coding categories rather than exploration of latent meanings. Deductive codes were adopted from Lovejoy and Saxton's (2012) study of how non-profit organizations use social media to leverage followers and drive advocacy campaigns online. In all, twelve sub-categories of tweets were identified from Lovejoy and Saxton (2012), representing three meta-categories: information-oriented tweets, community-building tweets, and action-oriented tweets. Information-oriented content provides community members and supporters with timely updates on latest developments, patient challenges, and disease-specific news. Community-building content aims to socialize members and strengthen interpersonal ties within the community. Action-oriented content concerns mobilizing community members to take supportive actions towards achieving campaign goals. In many cases, tweet content related to more than one category and therefore was dual-coded for richness[15] (see Figures 4.1 and 4.2 for a breakdown). In addition, we measured the frequency of tweet behavior and the sequencing of tweet behavior across both campaigns.

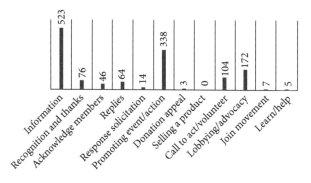

Figure 4.1 Tweet categories by @YesOrkambi
Note: Some tweets belong to more than one topic category

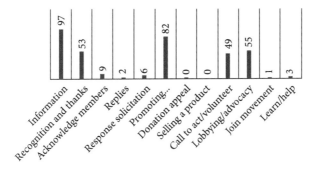

Figure 4.2 Tweet categories by @SMAIrelandCom
Note: Some tweets belong to more than one topic category

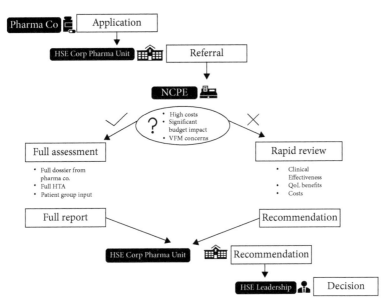

Figure 4.3 The assessment process for drug reimbursement in Ireland
Note: HSE: Health Services Executive; HTA: health technology assessment; NCPE: National Centre for Pharmacoeconomics Evaluation; QoL: quality of life; VFM: value for money

2.4 Study Context: The Assessment Process

Figure 4.3 maps the Irish assessment and approval process—in effect, the process by which the value of a drug is decided. When the HSE receives an application from a pharmaceutical company, its corporate pharmaceutical unit must commission the NCPE to conduct a health technology assessment

(HTA).[16] This includes a rapid review of the drug's regulatory status, the clinical condition targeted, the disease it should be licensed for, how the drug will fit with current therapies, comparator or competitor drugs or therapies, clinical evidence, safety, efficacy, and economic considerations. The NCPE review concludes within four weeks and determines whether a full pharmacoeconomic assessment is required. High-cost products, those with significant budget impact, or products where concerns arise in relation to value for money must undergo formal pharmacoeconomic assessment in a full HTA. Here the drug manufacturer is asked to detail the health economics and incremental benefits that justify the drug's increased cost, and submissions by patient groups are facilitated.

All drug assessments (orphan drugs included) are carried out in compliance with guidelines published by the Health Information and Quality Authority (HIQA). HIQA points out that Ireland's health budget is not unlimited and that investing in a particular drug may result in another health technology or service being dropped: "To make that choice, it is important that accurate and reliable evidence is presented to support decision-making. The goal of HTA is to provide that independent evidence."[17] The NCPE considers clinical effectiveness, quality-of-life benefits, and all relevant costs including potential savings such as lower use of other healthcare resources (e.g. hospital beds) to judge whether the price quoted by the manufacturer is justified. The NCPE then advises the HSE on the value for money and budget impact of the drug. The full assessment report, any commercial negotiations, and other relevant information are considered by the HSE drugs group, which makes a recommendation to the HSE leadership team as the final decision-making body. The 2013 Act provides no distinct assessment criteria for orphan drugs.

In Section 3 we present findings from two case studies of how the Irish approval process, designed to remove decision making from the political realm to ensure scientific objectivity, was influenced by a small group of active patients using social media to inform, activate, and mobilize support for their causes.

3. Influence and Decision Making in Ireland's Drug Reimbursement Process

3.1 The YesOrkambi Campaign

The patient-led, social media-based YesOrkambi campaign posted frequently on Twitter in an attempt to overturn the initial Orkambi reimbursement refusal. Campaign tactics included publicizing personalized patient experiences of life with CF, highlighting success stories of those on Orkambi trials, and lobbying local representatives and national government, all reinforced by the hashtag #YesOrkambi. This campaign started strongly, generating 10 percent of its total tweet count in the first month of campaigning— communicating both the seriousness and urgency behind the campaign. In November–December 2016, we see a spike in tweets in conjunction with offline demonstrations and protest marches outside the Dáil in response to the HSE's second Orkambi reimbursement refusal. Such coordinated activities proved fruitful as price negotiations reopened between the HSE and Vertex Pharmaceuticals in December 2016 and continued into 2017. After a slow start to 2017, the YesOrkambi campaign ratcheted up advocacy activity once again in February when supporters engaged in joint online/offline candlelight vigils, tweeting photos along with the hashtags #YesOrkambi and #CFLivesMatter. These efforts were sustained into March 2017 where once again Twitter activity spiked in line with the campaign's second Dáil demonstration. A timeline of key campaign events is outlined in Figure 4.4.

Orkambi was approved for reimbursement in April 2017; since then there has been very little activity on the YesOrkambi Twitter account. The advocacy campaign had effectively achieved its aim. We analyze the role of social media in facilitating the YesOrkambi advocacy campaign across twelve content categories representing three advocacy dimensions of communicating with the community, connecting with politicians, and leveraging the media (Lovejoy and Saxton 2012).

3.1.1 The Role of Social Media in YesOrkambi

The YesOrkambi campaign splits its efforts quite evenly between providing members with information (51.58 percent of tweets) and rallying for action (50.20 percent of tweets). It devoted much less time to community-building efforts (19.37 percent of tweets). This is perhaps due to the presence of a pre-existing patient community, as people with CF are already well connected through the CFI network. Therefore, it may have been deemed less necessary to socialize members to the purpose of the advocacy campaign than to share important new information and updates, or to organize the campaign's social actions. Information-oriented tweets in this context largely consisted of providing community members with commentary and updates on progress, or lack thereof, in price negotiations, as well as highlighting individual patient experiences with CF. Within the action-oriented tweets disseminated by YesOrkambi, three action topic categories accounted for the majority of this

98 "PLEASE DON'T PUT A PRICE ON OUR LIVES"

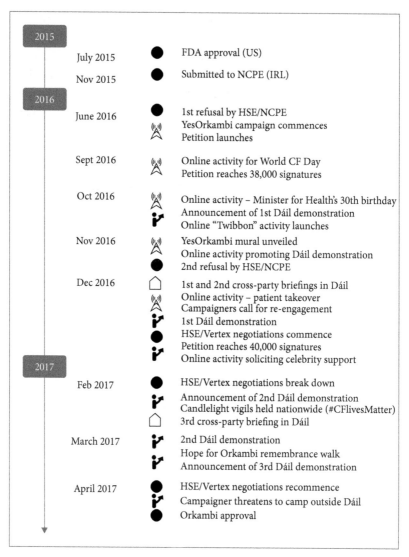

Figure 4.4 Timeline of key YesOrkambi campaign highlights

activity: (1) promoting an event/action (for instance a Dáil demonstration) (66.5 percent of all of action-oriented tweets); (2) lobbying/advocacy activities specifically directed at other market actors (33.86 percent of action-oriented tweets); and (3) direct calls to act/volunteer aimed at mobilizing community members and supporters (20.47 percent of action-oriented tweets). Community-building efforts, while few, primarily concentrated on providing recognition and thanks to members and the wider public for their support, as well as replying to tweets posted by other members (over 70 percent of all community-building tweets).

From this analysis, YesOrkambi organizers undertook a sustained and coordinated advocacy campaign alongside supporting offline social actions such as Dáil demonstrations. This advocacy campaign balanced a largely two-pronged social media approach throughout, informing and mobilizing community members through posting information-oriented and action-oriented tweets. Unsurprisingly, there is an increase in information sharing and calls to action in the days prior to organized social actions (e.g. Dáil demonstrations), with a preponderance of action-oriented tweets on those days, and a return to information-oriented tweets in the days following social actions. In particular, information such as patient stories and media coverage are highlighted to supporters. Community-building tweets are peppered sporadically across the campaign timeline, providing multiple opportunities for campaign organizers to maintain support from the community and others.

Throughout the YesOrkambi advocacy campaign we see a concerted effort by campaign organizers and their supporters to politicize their drug reimbursement issue through frequent references to, and direct engagement with, various actors including the government, specific government ministers (minster for health, minister for finance, etc.), the HSE, NCPE, and Vertex Pharmaceuticals. YesOrkambi campaigners use Twitter effectively to confront government politicians and other actors, challenging their perceived complacency/inaction over the drug pricing and reimbursement approval process at the heart of this advocacy campaign. In the first instance, social media permit YesOrkambi advocates to follow and respond to updates from politicians and decision makers, engaging them in dialogue to further the YesOrkambi cause. This feeds into information-oriented tweets where updates are circulated to community members. Replying to politicians, the HSE or Vertex enables campaigners to seek direct clarification and follow up information in the interest of the patient community.

Advocates for YesOrkambi regularly "call out" perceived political complacency by highlighting the length of time elapsed since Orkambi's initial refusal, and the lack of progress in the interim—but also offering their willingness to engage in the process. For example: "It's over 14 weeks. Can anyone give us a timeline? What can we do to help! #YesOrkambi @VertexPharma @SimonHarrisTD."[18] Such campaign tweets publicly demand increased accountability from those in power while helping to maintain momentum in the advocacy campaign. They accentuate the plight of the patients and reinforce the urgency of their cause: "We're not going anywhere. 23 weeks is just so wrong. @VertexPharma & @HSElive there are lives caught in the middle. It's cruel. #YesOrkambi." The minister for health is a particular target for such confrontational challenges. Through retweeting behaviors, YesOrkambi campaigners further draw attention to certain political activities such as highlighting mentions of Orkambi and campaign actions in the Dáil. They thank and recognize members of the opposition for elevating their cause in these political forums, as well as for offering their personal support at organized demonstrations and other events. As this support grows, more pressure is exerted on the decision makers to come to a resolution. A timeline indicating key political actions highlighted by the YesOrkambi campaign is outlined in Figure 4.5.

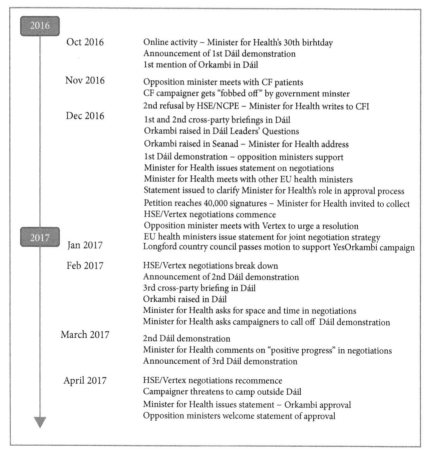

Figure 4.5 Timeline of key political actions highlighted by YesOrkambi

Through social media, YesOrkambi campaigners also engage with the mainstream media to heighten their advocacy campaign in the public consciousness. Several prominent YesOrkambi advocates undertake mass media activities and participate in public debates in local and national newspapers, on national news and current affairs television programs, as well as on the radio. They give interviews, write op-ed articles, and share their stories. They engage in dialogue with journalists on Twitter, willingly offering their time and experiences for publication. YesOrkambi supporters and campaign organizers readily share and retweet these articles, video clips, and podcasts across social media to broadcast them widely and promote the mass media coverage afforded to the advocacy campaign. Through Twitter, campaigners also acknowledge and thank the media for their support. We see a significant increase in media coverage, and supporter broadcasting of the same, in the two weeks prior to the first YesOrkambi Dáil demonstration on December 7, 2016, which strengthens the campaign's calls for more decisive action to be taken on all sides. As the demonstration, and its media coverage, gets under way, the mass media also breaks news of the decision by the HSE and Vertex Pharmaceutical to recommence drug-pricing talks with renewed hope for reaching an agreement.

3.2 The SpinrazaNow Campaign

Figure 4.6 outlines the ebb and flow of the Spinraza reimbursement advocacy campaign. The SpinrazaNow campaign launched nine months after the NCPE's recommendation to refuse reimbursement in December 2017, and more than a year after its submission to the NCPE for approval in July 2017. The delayed launch appears to have afforded the SpinrazaNow organizers and their supporters an opportunity to strategize so that their campaign could be as effective as possible. On social media, SMAIrelandCom drove the SpinrazaNow advocacy campaign. Alongside the campaign launched on Twitter, organizers also launched a dedicated campaign website, SMAIreland. com, to provide more detailed information to the patient community, as well as to create a patient database and to communicate with interested parties around how to get involved in its advocacy efforts. For instance, it provided guidelines and a template for joining in with its social media video campaign, along with contact details for advocating directly to decision makers (e.g. Minister for Health, local councilors, HSE, etc.).

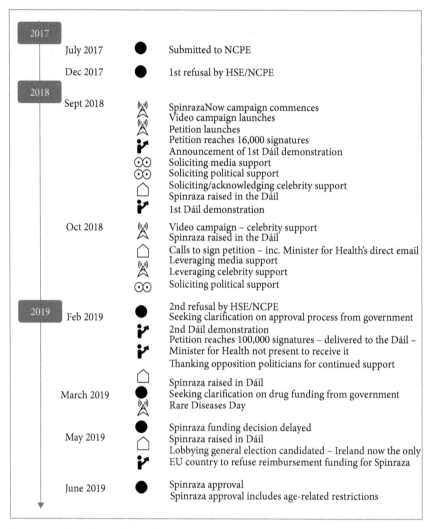

Figure 4.6 Timeline of key SpinrazaNow campaign and political highlights

Twitter activity across the SpinrazaNow campaign was less frequent and more sporadic than that of YesOrkambi, generating approximately 75 percent fewer tweets in total—just 247 tweets compared to YesOrkambi's 1,012 tweets. Following a relatively strong start to campaigning and a spike in Twitter activity, there is a significant drop off in online posting and during some months no online activity at all. Furthermore, we do not see the same intensity in tweeting behavior at pivotal points during this ten-month campaign, as peaks and troughs are much less pronounced. Nevertheless, this advocacy campaign was highly effective in focusing on the key reimbursement issue and drawing in a large supporter base collectively throwing its significant weight and influence behind the SpinrazaNow campaign.

3.2.1 The Role of Social Media in SpinrazaNow

In addition to its delayed start, the SpinrazaNow advocacy campaign took a very different direction to YesOrkambi from the outset. SMAIrelandCom was instantly more focused on using social media to rally its community members into action. Over two-thirds of all tweets posted across this campaign were action-oriented (68.04 percent), while 44.27 percent of tweets were information-oriented. Less than one-third (31.51 percent) of SMAIrelandCom's tweets were concerned with community-building efforts. Again, this may have been intentional given the small size of this patient community, just twenty-five children across the country. It is likely that this patient group already formed a tight-knit support community prior to the launch of this advocacy campaign. Similar to YesOrkambi, this would negate the necessity of spending time cultivating patient support and informing them of the purpose of the advocacy campaign (Lovejoy and Saxton 2012). Instead, information-oriented tweets were focused on sharing insights into patient challenges and updates on Spinraza's effectiveness.

The SpinrazaNow Twitter campaign adopted a concerted action-oriented approach by immediately promoting community action from its very first tweet. One of this campaign's defining characteristics was the seeking out of supporters with influence (e.g. Irish sports stars and celebrities) to tweet on its behalf to raise greater awareness. Campaign organizers provided supporters with online templates and advice on how to create advocacy messages and supporting videos to share with their social networks across social media. This approach resulted in over 55 percent of all action-oriented tweets specifically focusing on promoting a variety of key campaign events and actions. In addition, almost one-third (32.88 percent) of action-oriented tweets also included a direct call to act, designed to encourage more supporters to get involved in campaigning efforts. Furthermore, 36.91 percent of all action-oriented tweets involved lobbying and advocacy efforts explicitly aimed at state and corporate market actors.

In terms of community-building efforts, SpinrazaNow campaign tweets largely consisted of recognizing and thanking those who participated in the advocacy campaign (76.81 percent of all community-related tweets). In particular, gratitude was extended to celebrities and others for their support, thus further amplifying this support while encouraging others to get involved through embedding specific calls to act. As such, a number of community-building tweets were also considered action-oriented tweets as campaign organizers adopted a dual purpose in showing their appreciation and recognition of community members and supporters.

The SpinrazaNow advocacy campaign adopted by SMAIrelandCom appeared to follow a clear strategic intent, perhaps due to learnings gained from the YesOrkambi campaign that had taken place a year earlier. The YesOrkambi campaign favored a dual-orientation approach, balancing information- and action-oriented tweets (51.68 and 50.20 percent, respectively). YesOrkambi focused much less on community-building activities than SpinrazaNow (19.37 versus 31.51 percent); however, it did have a much higher incidence of replying to tweets from members and others to acknowledge their campaign involvement. In contrast, SMAIrelandCom concentrated on sharing action-oriented bite-sized content with followers to encourage their engagement and advocacy support (68.04 percent). In fact, the SpinrazaNow campaign included a direct call to action in 22.37 percent of tweets, compared to just 10.28 percent of YesOrkambi's tweets. In addition, the lobbying/advocacy efforts of SpinrazaNow were proportionally much greater than those of YesOrkambi, at 25.11 percent and 17 percent, respectively (Figure 4.7). Perhaps this reflected a lesson learned from the earlier YesOrkambi campaign, which empowered SMAIrelandCom to be more forthright in its social media campaigning for SpinrazaNow.

Throughout the SpinrazaNow advocacy campaign, we notice a distinct politically focused activity not evident in the YesOrkambi campaign—direct solicitation of politicians requesting their support in securing funding for Spinraza in Ireland. SMAIrelandCom and SpinrazaNow supporters frequently tweeted government ministers and local councilors, as well as Irish ministers of European Parliament and presidential candidates asking them to engage with the advocacy campaign's efforts by attending events (e.g. Dáil demonstrations) or signing a petition, amongst others. Campaigners lobbied politicians by tweeting them directly to seek their support, exploiting the platform

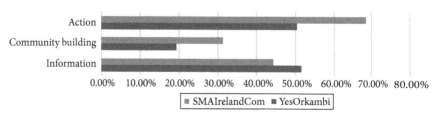

Figure 4.7 Comparison of tweet categories

Note: The figures do not add to 100 percent as some tweets belong to more than one topic category

architecture of Twitter to bring this advocacy campaign in front of powerful actors and decision makers. Social media solicitation is an activity that recurs throughout this campaign.

For those politicians who do engage, for example by raising the case for Spinraza in the Dáil or by creating advocacy videos as part of the social media SpinrazaNow video campaign, SMAIrelandCom retweeted this information in order to acknowledge, show appreciation for, and amplify political support. Similar to YesOrkambi, broadcasting political backing bolstered the SpinrazaNow advocacy campaign by signaling a growing support, and therefore strength, behind the campaign. As more members of the opposition get involved, their clout gives credence to the campaign's demands, and again raises the issue of drug-pricing reimbursement in broader civic and public domains.

In addition, the SpinrazaNow campaign actively used Twitter to denounce perceived political complacency in relation to the reimbursement of drug funding. Campaign organizers launched and frequently promoted links to a petition to bring this issue to the steps of Dáil and collected in excess of 100,000 signatures along the way by leveraging supporter networks across social media. Moreover, SpinrazaNow campaigners took to Twitter to vent their frustration when Ireland became the only outstanding country in the European Union not to reimburse funding for the Spinraza drug. Going further than YesOrkambi, SpinrazaNow campaigners called on their social networks to avoid voting for present government ministers in national elections running during the campaign's time frame. In all, social media was crucial to initiating and sustaining political pressure for the SpinrazaNow campaign.

SMAIrelandCom also used social media to solicit support and coverage from the mainstream media. Through actions such as tweeting journalists and current affairs programs, SMAIrelandCom and SpinrazaNow advocates offered interviews and appearances to bring wider attention to their cause, for instance: "Willing to talk to anyone who will listen.. community groups, media. This morning our [campaigner] left [local] church in silence when she addressed them. THANK YOU for taking time to listen and help #SpinrazaNOW @RyanTubridyShow @joeliveline." Such online actions were particularly evident in the days leading up to Dáil demonstrations in an effort to create as much advocacy "noise" as possible in order to draw attention to the campaign, for example: "@ghook Be great to have your coverage of #SpinrazaNOW campaign for SMA sufferers in Ireland. We're coming to Dublin on Thursday."

Coverage gained by mass media outlets was publicly acknowledged and appreciated on social media by the SpinrazaNow campaigners. Retweeting of news articles and video/audio clips helped to amplify the mass media's coverage and encouraged more media support for the advocacy campaign. The importance of mass media coverage was clearly understood by the SpinrazaNow campaign organizers as having the potential to refocus public awareness of and support for funding Spinraza. This leveraging of mass media support is reminiscent of the approach adopted by the YesOrkambi advocacy campaign a year earlier.

Lastly, SpinrazaNow campaigners also solicited the support of Irish celebrities and sports stars via social media. Individuals who participated in the SpinrazaNow video campaign (calling for funding using a refined video template/script issued by SMAIrelandCom) were recognized and thanked for their support. Again, leveraging this support through tweets and retweets helped to amplify the SpinrazaNow campaign message while reaching vast secondary audiences consisting of all those following these well-known Irish stars on social media (Kaplan and Haenlein 2010). Similar to leveraging mass media coverage, leveraging celebrity support also helped bring the campaign for Spinraza funding into the limelight, drawing public attention towards this issue. This added publicity reinvigorated and emboldened campaigners to continue to advocate for Spinraza.

4. The Multiple Roles of Social Media in Healthcare Activism

4.1 Social Media Enroll New Actors

Social media enroll other media in the debate. Much of the social media literature speaks of social media as "open access" platforms (Hoffman and Novak 1996, 51), implying an open door through which interested others can gain access to the campaign. Our data show a less passive role for social media in the campaign. Our social media campaigns actively reach out and enroll others within, including mainstream media and celebrities. Although it is a small sample of only two cases, our data appear to indicate an increasing use of social media to perform such active enrolment within the healthcare market in Ireland, with the Spinraza campaign exceeding the Orkambi campaign in this regard.

In our data we see the campaigns, particularly that of SMAIrelandCom, reaching out to mainstream media and weaving mainstream and social media narratives together to reinforce the campaign. Mainstream media must, to a certain extent, maintain an objective presence "above the fray," so to speak. It has checks and balances in terms of editorial policies and verification processes. Social media have no such limits and facilitates pure advocacy "to further or achieve specific policy goals" as outlined by Obar et al. (2012, 4). Our cases demonstrate how social media are used to harness the apparent objectivity of the mass media and utilize this in the social media campaign. The moral authority and public trust that is conferred by the direct patient voice bearing witness to their struggles (McDonnell 2016) is exponentially strengthened by the apparent objective endorsement of the mass media.

The mass media are not the only "other" to be enrolled by social media. The Spinraza case also demonstrates the recruitment of celebrities and sports stars in support of the SpinrazaNow campaign. These celebrities are used to amplify the calls and claims of the campaign as their social influence is harnessed via the social media campaign. This not only lends weight to campaign statements in the form of endorsement, it also extends the campaign as those who follow these celebrities become aware of, and active in, the campaign. This is seen in the dual coding of a number of our case tweets that refer to celebrities as both community building and action-oriented, where the social media campaign organizers extended thanks to, and highlighted the actions of, these enrolled celebrities. These celebrities are neither similar to (Tajfel 1978) nor more knowledgeable or experienced than (McAlexander et al. 2002) the patient advocates who are behind the social media campaigns. This therefore extends the previous view of patient-led advocacy campaigns that use social networking sites. While our cases do, as previously catalogued, present patients' own personalized experiences and struggles (Penney 2015; Yang 2016), they go beyond this to enroll and mobilize non-patient influencers in the campaign.

4.2 Social Media Mobilize Actors Offline

Beyond that, social media act as coordinating tools for offline action. The social media literature builds a strong case for the role of social media in creating patient communities within healthcare (Obar et al. 2012; Zuckerman 2014; Penney 2015; Housley et al. 2018). The literature describes how healthcare has become more subject to market culture and how actors can act to shape that market. Our research demonstrates that certain social media campaigns actually spend little time or effort on community building amongst the patient community but rather focus on the provision of information and rallying for action. In the timelines presented in our findings above (Figures 4.4, 4.5, 4.6), the connection between online social media activities and offline activities such as marches, vigils, and petitions is clear. Social media campaigns are used to publicize these activities, facilitate engagement in the offline activities, and actively recruit existing and new actors to these offline activities. Post-fact, social media campaigns are used to amplify the offline activities, posting commentaries on or images from the relevant march or vigil.

4.3 Social Media Are Used to Challenge Powerful Actors

The platform architecture of Twitter facilitates users to connect, follow, and address others without the need for reciprocation, a unique feature among most social media sites. Such a feature assists campaigners and advocates coming into direct contact with power holders and decision makers, a difficult feat under other circumstances. Both cases demonstrate how social media are used to solicit, criticize, confront, or question various actors including the government, specific government ministers (Minster for Health, Minister for Finance, etc.), the HSE, NCPE, and Big Pharma. Social media are used to hold such actors accountable and question their definitions of value. As such, social media facilitate patient voices more readily entering the market approval process, which so markedly affects them. Social media strengthen patient voices in their criticism of actors involved in the approval process. Moreover, community advocates use social media to broadcast their appreciation for support gained from politicians. This encourages more supporters to get involved in campaigning and singles out those ministers who enable this process to continue.

These three roles are mutually reinforcing. The relationship between mass media and social media assists in the mobilization of actors as mass media publicize and subsequently report on offline protests and vigils. The mobilization of offline protests adds weight to the challenge of powerful actors—bringing the protest to their door both literally and metaphorically. Likewise, the challenging of powerful actors provides further fodder for mainstream media coverage and offers a focus point for offline action. Social media act as a thread that weaves these elements together so that they become a coordinated campaign. Figure 4.8 summarizes the roles and impact of social media.

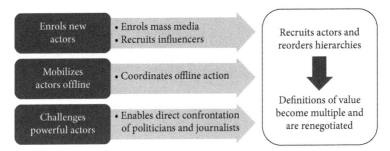

Figure 4.8 The roles and impact of social media within healthcare

4.4 Social Media Extend the Community and Definitions of Value Are Renegotiated

As the mass media become involved in the market the number of people participating in the issue snowballs. This is particularly evident in the Spinraza case where the initial affected public extended to just twenty-five children and their families. By the end of the social media campaign, hundreds of new advocates supported the call for SpinrazaNow. This new weight of supporters, combined with the ability to tackle powerful actors such as government and "Big Pharma" in a public arena, generates greater "noise" and elevates the issue of drug pricing and reimbursement from a market challenge to a larger societal issue. In doing so, a two-way influence is forged between the market and wider society—social media bring market-specific concerns into the public domain, and societal concerns must be dealt with at the market level. These concerns challenge the legislation-based method of defining value within the market. Throughout the legislative rule-based process, information as to value is provided based on the probability of cost-effectiveness at a range of thresholds. For example, a value is placed on the quality adjustment per year of a patient's life on the drug in ranges: €20,000 per quality adjusted life year (QALY); €45,000 per QALY; and €100,000 per QALY. As the title of this chapter suggests, however, social media advocacy campaigns seek to change the definition of value that underpins current market rules asking that legislators and decision makers "do not put a value on our lives." However, in both of our cases these changes in value definition appear somewhat time-bound and last only as long as the advocacy campaigns themselves. Despite efforts to introduce changes to the drug reimbursement legislation on the back of such campaigns, no real policy changes have been implemented. An amendment to the Health Act (2013), raised in 2018, proposed "a threshold cost-effective incremental ratio or similar assessment, shall not be relevant in the case of Orphan Medicinal Products."[19] Yet as of January 14, 2020 this proposed amendment to the Health Act (2013) has now lapsed, and no such changes have been enacted.[20]

Conclusion

We set out to examine how social media campaigns might affect drug reimbursement in Ireland in the particular case of two orphan drugs. Our data suggest that social media play three key, interrelated roles within that context—enrolling new actors, challenging powerful actors, and mobilizing offline action. Together these three roles combine to extend the range of actors involved and introduce societal concerns into the economic evaluation process. This in turn opens up new discussions as to what constitutes value that challenge existing definitions of value within healthcare. We offer indicative findings and thoughts as to the role of social media in healthcare that raise more questions as to the complementary or contradictory roles that mass media and other actors may play alongside social media. We therefore suggest that future research examine the intersection between mainstream media, social media, and legislative action in shaping value in healthcare to better understand the relationships between all three.

In addition to contesting definitions of value by enrolling and mobilizing new actors, social media have produced a further outcome in the power dynamics of market actors. Social media activism shone a spotlight on the orphan drug reimbursement process and the economic assessment of value underlying it. By challenging public discourse on what constitutes value through social media activism, patient communities in essence have served to strengthen the hand of "Big Pharma"—arguably already the most powerful player in this market. Through demanding access to orphan drugs, patient influence has gone further to instigate a change in altering the process for calculating value in terms of orphan drug cost-effectiveness. Bill 33 of 2018, the amendment to the Health Act (2013), seeks to remove the government's right to question the objective cost-effectiveness of orphan drugs prior to their reimbursement. Should this Bill pass through the Irish Parliament (Dáil), it would undoubtedly benefit patients, yet it would also serve to line the pockets of drug manufacturers who would face less scrutiny. Here the enrolment of patient communities into the reimbursement process arguably leverages the weakest market player to do the bidding of the most powerful. This raises the question as to which market actors benefit most from social media-led activism campaigns.

The global pharmaceutical market is reliant on orphan drugs for much of its predicted future expansion. Between 2018 and 2024, orphan drugs are expected to outperform the market, accounting for 20 percent of total prescription drug sales and forecast to almost double in size to $262 billion in 2024. One industry report comments that this reflects the pharmaceutical industry's focus on "small groups of neglected patients with high unmet need and to benefit from traditionally reduced payer scrutiny on orphan drugs, as well as regulatory and financial incentives" (Evaluate Pharma 2018, 8). It is these two points—the high unmet need of the patient and the review and negotiation of drug prices, that form the basis of our cases. These counterpoints mean that although there is great promise in new therapies that successfully treat the rarest of diseases for the smallest patient populations, market processes, and particularly approaches to pricing and reimbursement, must keep pace with pharmaceutical innovation in order to ensure access, equity, and sustainability of supply—in short, to reconcile market and civic logics within the provision of orphan drugs. "The promise of these new therapies will only become reality if the innovation of drug companies is matched by innovation in the drug pricing and reimbursement systems" (Evaluate Pharma 2019).

Acknowledgments

The researchers would like to gratefully acknowledge funding received from the Donnellan Fund, Maynooth University School of Business in supporting this research.

Notes

1. RTE News, June 11, 2019, https://www.rte.ie/news/health/2019/0611/1054770-spinraza-drug/, accessed August 9, 2019.
2. Professor Michael Barry, Director of the National Centre for Pharmacoeconomics, addressing the 2018 Irish Medical Organisation AGM.
3. Roche, Barry, Ireland Should Lead in Cystic Fibrosis Care, Says Consultant, *The Irish Times*, March 31, 2017.
4. The Cystic Fibrosis Registry of Ireland, Annual Report, 2017, https://www.cfri.ie/docs/annual_reports/CFRI2017.pdf, accessed May 9, 2019.
5. Cystic Fibrosis Ireland website, https://www.cfireland.ie/about-cf, accessed May 9, 2019.

112 "PLEASE DON'T PUT A PRICE ON OUR LIVES"

6. https://www.thejournal.ie/spinraza-sma-hse-4512136-Feb2019/, accessed February 24, 2020.
7. https://www.curesma.org/type-of-sma/, accessed February 24, 2020.
8. Spinal Muscular Atrophy Ireland Website, http://smaireland.com/about-sma-spinal-muscular-atrophy/, accessed June 11, 2019.
9. European Medicines Agency, EMA/736370/2017 EMEA/H/C/004312 EPAR summary for the public, Spinraza, https://www.ema.europa.eu/en/documents/overview/spinraza-epar-summary-public_en.pdf, accessed June 11, 2016.
10. Pre-submission consultation with applicant September 12, 2017, submission received from applicant October 31, 2017, preliminary review sent to applicant November 28, 2017, NCPE assessment recommenced December 6, 2017, applicant factual accuracy check December 8, 2017, NCPE assessment recommenced December 14, 2017.
11. https://www.thejournal.ie/spinraza-sma-hse-4512136-Feb2019/, accessed February 24, 2020.
12. https://rothco.ie/news/you-pick-on-one-of-us-you-pick-on-all-of-us/, accessed February 21, 2020.
13. https://twitter.com/YesOrkambi, accessed February 25, 2020.
14. http://smaireland.com/spinrazanow-campaign/, accessed February 25, 2020.
15. Note that numbers/percentages cited for social media statistics do not add to 100 percent as some tweets belong to more than one topic category.
16. A health technology assessment employs a multi-disciplinary research process to collect and summarize information about a health technology including clinical effectiveness and safety, cost-effectiveness and budget impact, organizational and social aspects, and ethical and legal issues that is collected and presented in a systematic, unbiased, and transparent manner.
17. HIQA website, https://www.hiqa.ie/areas-we-work/health-technology-assessment, accessed September 2, 2019.
18. Simon Harris was Minister for Health at the time of this tweet.
19. Professor Michael Barry, Director of the National Centre for Pharmacoeconomics, addressing the 2018 Irish Medical Organisation AGM.
20. Health (Pricing and Supply of Medical Goods) (Amendment) Bill 2018 https://www.oireachtas.ie/en/bills/bill/2018/33/.

References

Abraham, J. (2009), The Pharmaceutical Industry, the State and the NHS, in J. Gabe and M. Calnan (eds) *The New Sociology of the Health Service*, London: Routledge.

Acerete, B., Stafford, A., and Stapleton, P. (2012), New Development: New Global Health Care PPP Developments: A Critique of the Success Story. *Public Money and Management*, 32:4, 311–14.

Acosta, R. (2012), Advocacy Networks through a Multidisciplinary Lens: Implications for Research Agendas, *VOLUNTAS: International Journal of Voluntary and Nonprofit Organizations*, 23:1, 156–81.

Ahrne, G., Aspers, P., and Brunsson, N. (2015), The Organization of Markets, *Organization Studies*, 36:1, 7–27.

Attai, D. J., Cowher, M. S., Al-Hamadani, M., Schoger, J. M., Staley, A. C., and Landercasper, J. (2015), Twitter Social Media Is an Effective Tool for Breast Cancer Patient Education and Support: Patient-Reported Outcomes by Survey, *Journal of Medical Internet Research*, 17:7, e188.

Bagozzi, R. P., and Dholakia, U. M. (2002), Intentional Social Action in Virtual Communities, *Journal of Interactive Marketing*, 16:2, 2–21.

Berger, J., and Milkman, K. L. (2012), What Makes Online Content Viral? *Journal of Marketing Research*, 49:2, 192–205.

Burgel, P.-R., Bellis, G., Olesen, H. V., Viviani, L., Zolin, A., Blasi, F., and Elborn, J. S. (2015), Future Trends in Cystic Fibrosis Demography in 34 European Countries, *European Respiratory Journal*, 46, 133–41.

Dacin, M. T., Ventresca, M. J., and Beal, B. D. (1999), The Embeddedness of Organizations: Dialogue and Directions, *Journal of Management*, 25:3, 317–56.

Dholakia, U. M., Bagozzi, R. P., and Pearo, L. K. (2004), A Social Influence Model of Consumer Participation in Network-and Small-Group-Based Virtual Communities, *International Journal of Research in Marketing*, 21:3, 241–63.

Djelic, M. L. (2012), Scholars in the Audit Society: Understanding Our Contemporary Iron Cage, in *Scholars in Action Past-Present-Future*, Edita Västra Aros, Lars Engwall, 97–121.

Djelic, M. L., and Sahlin-Andersson, K. (eds) (2006), *Transnational Governance: Institutional Dynamics of Regulation*, Cambridge University Press.

Dubuisson-Quellier, S. (2013), A Market Mediation Strategy: How Social Movements Seek to Change Firms' Practices by Promoting New Principles of Product Valuation, *Organization Studies*, 34:5–6, 683–703.

Eikenberry, A. M., and Kluver, J. D. (2004), The Marketization of the Nonprofit Sector: Civil Society at Risk? *Public Administration Review*, 64:2, 132–40.

Eisenhardt, K. M. (1989), Building Theories from Case Study Research, *Academy of Management Review*, 14:4, 532–50.

Evaluate Pharma (2018), World Preview 2018, Outlook to 2023, 11th Edition, June.

Evaluate Pharma (2019), Orphan Drug Report 2019, 6th Edition, April.

Fundación Bamberg (2011), El modelo de future de gestión de la salud. Available at: http://fundacionbamberg.org/actualidad/noticias/coincidiendo-con-25-aniversario-ley-generalsanidad-fundacion-bamberg-presenta-m

Geiger, S., Harrison, D., Kjellberg, H., and Mallard, A. (2014), Being Concerned about Markets, in S. Geiger, D. Harrison, H. Kjellberg, and A. Mallard (eds), *Concerned Markets*, Edward Elgar Publishing.

Giroux, H. A. (2004), Public Pedagogy and the Politics of Neo-Liberalism: Making the Political More Pedagogical, *Policy Futures in Education*, 2:3–4, 494–503.

Hajer, M. A. (1995), *The Politics of Environmental Discourse: Ecological Modernization and the Policy Process*, Oxford: Clarendon Press.

Hauser, G. A. (1999), *Vernacular Voices: The Rhetoric of Publics and Public Spheres*, University of South Carolina Press.

Hewett, K., Rand, W., Rust, R. T., and Van Heerde, H. J. (2016), Brand Buzz in the Echoverse, *Journal of Marketing*, 80:3, 1–24.

Hoffman, A. J. (1999), Institutional Evolution and Change: Environmentalism and the US Chemical Industry, *Academy of Management Journal*, 42:4, 351–71.

Hoffman, D. L., and Novak, T. P. (1996), Marketing in Hypermedia Computer-Mediated Environments: Conceptual Foundations, *Journal of Marketing*, 60:3, 50–68.

Housley, W., Webb, H., Williams, M., Procter, R., Edwards, A., Jirotka, M. et al. (2018), Interaction and Transformation on Social Media: The Case of Twitter Campaigns, *Social Media+ Society*, 4:1, 1–12.

Johnen, M., Jungblut, M., and Ziegele, M. (2018), The Digital Outcry: What Incites Participation Behavior in an Online Firestorm? *New Media and Society*, 20:9, 3140–60.

Kaplan, A. M., and Haenlein, M. (2010), Users of the World, Unite! The Challenges and Opportunities of Social Media, *Business Horizons*, 53:1, 59–68.

Kraemer, R., Whiteman, G., and Banerjee, B. (2013), Conflict and Astroturfing in Niyamgiri: The Importance of National Advocacy Networks in Anti-Corporate Social Movements, *Organization Studies*, 34:5–6, 823–52.

Krippendorff, K. (2013), *Content Analysis: An Introduction to Its Methodology* (2nd edition), London: Sage.

Lovejoy, K., and Saxton, G. D. (2012), Information, Community, and Action: How Nonprofit Organizations Use Social Media, *Journal of Computer-Mediated Communication*, 17:3, 337–53.

McAlexander, J. H., Schouten, J. W., and Koenig, H. F. (2002), Building Brand Community, *Journal of Marketing*, 66:1, 38–54.

McDonnell, M. H. (2016), Radical Repertoires: The Incidence and Impact of Corporate-Sponsored Social Activism, *Organization Science*, 27:1, 53–71.

Meng, J., Peng, W., Tan, P. N., Liu, W., Cheng, Y., and Bae, A. (2018), Diffusion Size and Structural Virality: The Effects of Message and Network Features on Spreading Health Information on Twitter, *Computers in Human Behavior*, 89, 111–20.

Moran, G., Muzellec, L., and Johnson, D. (2019), Message Content Features and Social Media Engagement: Evidence from the Media Industry, *Journal of Product and Brand Management*, doi.org/10.1108/JPBM-09-2018-2014

Mountford, N. (2019), Managing by Proxy: Organizational Networks as Institutional Levers in Evolving Public Good Markets, *Journal of Business Research*, 98, 92–104.

Mountford, N., and Geiger, S. (2020), Duos and Duels in Field Evolution: How Governments and Interorganizational Networks Relate, *Organization Studies*, 41:4, 499–522.

Murthy, D. (2018), Introduction to Social Media, Activism and Organizations, *Social Media + Society*, 4:1, 1–4.

Novas, C. (2009), Orphan Drugs, Patient Activism and Contemporary Healthcare, *Quaderni. Communication, technologies, pouvoir*, 68, 13–23.

Obar, J. A., Zube, P., and Lampe, C. (2012), Advocacy 2.0: An Analysis of How Advocacy Groups in the United States Perceive and Use Social Media as Tools for Facilitating Civic Engagement and Collective Action, *Journal of Information Policy*, 2, 1–25.

Penney, J. (2015), Social Media and Symbolic Action: Exploring Participation in the Facebook Red Equal Sign Profile Picture Campaign, *Journal of Computer-Mediated Communication*, 20, 52–66.

Poell, T., and Van Dijck, J. (2015), Social Media and Activist Communication, in *The Routledge Companion to Alternative and Community Media* (527–37), Routledge.

Rost, K., Stahel, L., and Frey, B. S. (2016), Digital Social Norm Enforcement: Online Firestorms in Social Media. *PLoS ONE*, 11:6, 1–26.

Smailhodzic, E., Hooijsma, W., Boonstra, A., and Langley, D. J. (2016), Social Media Use in Healthcare: A Systematic Review of Effects on Patients and on Their Relationship with Healthcare Professionals, *BMC Health Services Research*, 16:1, 442.

Soule, S. A. (2012), Social Movements and Markets, Industries, and Firms, *Organization Studies*, 33:12, 1715–33.

Tajfel, H. E. (1978), *Differentiation between Social Groups: Studies in the Social Psychology of Intergroup Relations*, Academic Press.

Thornton, P. H. (2002), The Rise of the Corporation in a Craft Industry: Conflict and Conformity in Institutional Logics, *Academy of Management Journal*, 45:1, 81–101.

Velasquez, A., and LaRose, R. (2015), Social Media for Social Change: Social Media Political Efficacy and Activism in Student Activist Groups, *Journal of Broadcasting and Electronic Media*, 59:3, 456–74.

Yang, G. (2016), Narrative Agency in Hashtag Activism: The Case of #BlackLivesMatter, *Media and Communication*, 4:4, 13.

Yin, R. K. (2014), *Case Study Research Design and Methods* (5th edition), Thousand Oaks, CA: Sage.

Zuckerman, E. (2014), New Media, New Civics? *Policy and Internet*, 6, 151–68.

5

Datafying the Patient Voice

The Making of Pervasive Infrastructures as Processes of Promise, Ruination, and Repair

Klaus Hoeyer and Henriette Langstrup

Introduction

Data have become objects of power struggles in multiple ways. It is increasingly through data that priorities are made, rankings established, and privileges granted or revoked (Erikson 2012; Kitchin 2014; Adams 2016; Merry 2016; Bigo et al. 2019). Data are tools of governance. Concurrently, new forms of activism are emerging around datafication where multiple parties try to influence what is datafied, by whom, for which purposes, and for whose sake. Rabeharisoa and colleagues identify in some of these data struggles a form of evidence-based activism, arguing that it involves a shift in positions: in contrast to classic notions of activism, this is done from within or in close collaboration with institutions rather than in opposition to them (Rabeharisoa et al. 2014). In evidence-based activism, data are mobilized as resources for collective action. It may involve datafication of patient voices: patient experiences are standardized and accumulated to allow organizations to speak on behalf of—or through the numbers of—populations, rather than through the narratives voiced by individuals. Who is seeking to datafy the patient voice, in which ways, and with which consequences? What do we learn about healthcare activism in an age of "intensified data sourcing" (Hoeyer 2016) from following the development of data infrastructures over time? These are bigger questions than can be answered in one chapter, but here we begin exploring them based on studies of infrastructural developments in Denmark.

Denmark is an interesting place to explore health data infrastructures and their intended and unintended consequences. The country is both a dedicated digital frontrunner and a pioneer in participatory methods, user-driven innovation, and citizen involvement in health technology assessments. In many

Klaus Hoeyer and Henriette Langstrup, *Datafying the Patient Voice: The Making of Pervasive Infrastructures as Processes of Promise, Ruination, and Repair* In: *Healthcare Activism: Markets, Morals, and the Collective Good.* Edited by: Susi Geiger, Oxford University Press. © Klaus Hoeyer and Henriette Langstrup 2021. DOI: 10.1093/oso/9780198865223.003.0005 ways, the country already has what many other countries only recently have begun to develop (Sheikh et al. 2015): nation-wide information technology infrastructures for health, decades of work with standard specification for exchange of health data, and a data infrastructure that since 1968 has ascribed traceable identity numbers to all individuals. Denmark is also a classic welfare state. Welfare states did not emerge out of nowhere: they are the result of enduring power struggles and contestation of rights and entitlements. Denmark has taken a route of what we call collaborative governance, by which we mean that the government generally seeks to contain and transform opposition rather than plainly suppress it. Whereas Mountford and Geiger (2018) describe specific strategies in collaborative governance that governments can adopt in relation to specific problems, we use the term here in a more general sense of governance that mostly seeks to establish consensus when dealing with contestations. Contestations thereby solidify into webs of legal frameworks as well as in various infrastructures aimed at creating opportunities for care as well as control.

Following Star and Ruhleder, we think of infrastructures as fundamentally relational: they are never finished and they have no clear boundaries (Star and Ruhleder 1996). Data infrastructures instantiate multiple historical layers of activism and means of governance. Gupta emphasizes the temporality of infrastructures: notwithstanding their accomplishments, they always carry the weight of failed promises of the past (Gupta 2018). In a sense, action in the present takes place in the ruins of infrastructures emanating out of promises made in the past. Jackson (2017) suggests considering this temporality as processes of breakdown, maintenance, and repair. Promises, however, precede the breakdown, and may survive in various ways without ever materializing as intended (Larkin 2013). The temporality is not linear. We think of ruination, not as total sojourn of function, but as processes where failures give rise to new forms of life and unintended uses (Tsing 2015). These spaces gradually emerge over time. With this inspiration, we approach infrastructuring as processes of *promise, ruination*, and *repair*. This understanding points to the need to understand the unfinished nature of activism. It also indicates an impossibility of delineating what and who are inside or outside a given infrastructure. Finally, it suggests a moral as well as epistemological ambiguity of the effect of power struggles.

In this chapter, we thus explore the multiple layers, unfinished nature, and unintended consequences of Danish data infrastructures for healthcare as intertwined processes of promise, ruination, and repair. We illustrate how government attempts at empowerment also involve examples of unintended

118 DATAFYING THE PATIENT VOICE

dis-empowerment and unwarranted vulnerabilities. Similarly, even the most well-intended and capable government attempts at empowerment can disappoint. Data integration is not without risk (O'Doherty et al. 2016). We also point to the way in which emerging data activism in the area of healthcare tends to give special voice to elitist groups. Our message is not pessimistic, however, as we wish to highlight all these attempts of repair as central to the continuous power struggles through which healthcare infrastructures take form and meet the needs of people confronted with illness and suffering.

1. How We Approach the Power Struggles of Datafication

As healthcare systems strive to become "data-driven" and "learning healthcare systems" (Olsen et al. 2007; Pollitt et al. 2010), power struggles and resource allocation issues increasingly unfold in relation to arguments based on available numbers (Wadmann et al. 2018; Hogle 2019). This datafication of health (Ruckenstein and Schüll 2017) also affects activism. The STS literature from the beginning of the twenty-first century on patient activism and health social movements (Epstein 1996; Brown et al. 2011; Wehling et al. 2014) drew to a large degree on a notion of activism as "spectacular political protest and opposition" against existing institutions and their "inadequate results and . . . unjust effects for certain groups of people and patients" (Wehling and Viehöver 2014, 240). In accordance with the popular image of the internet at the time as democratizing in its own right, patients' mobilization of digital means were often seen as instances of such authentic "voicing" and democratic empowerment (Slack 1997; Eysenbach 2001). In this chapter, we add to work exploring the shift to evidence-based patient activism by illustrating how the voicing of patients' concerns and perspectives by digital means need not take the form of *claimed spaces of protest* but increasingly means being part of *invited spaces of participation* (see also the chapter by Galasso and Geiger in this volume). According to Petersen and colleagues, datafication in itself can be said to have changed the nature of patient activism by enabling activist groups to use "the insights, expertise and financial support of science and corporations to achieve their goals" (Petersen et al. 2019, 23). Patient groups thus become more aligned with other mainstream actors, whether public or commercial, and more collaborative configurations or "hybrid forums" (Callon et al. 2002) emerge that may organize around shared concerns, which can challenge but also contribute to existing ways of knowing and governing. In a participation-oriented healthcare system like Denmark's, patient associations are valued collaborators—and "governing through participation" (Newman et al. 2004; Kjær and Pedersen 2010) has become the default also in relation to digitalization (Vikkelsø 2010).

In systems governed in such a collaborative manner, there is a need to remain skeptical toward equations of patient groups and activists. Opposition to mainstream versions of datafication of health often comes from quarters other than those organized around disease categories. This point is also supported in the emerging literature on "data activism," for which Lehtiniemi and Ruckenstein (2019) provide a number of recent examples in the context of health: in more and more instances, datafication is becoming an issue of political and civic action in its own right. Kennedy (2018) calls for more attention to "everyday data experience of datafication"—as opposed to spectacular protests and "elitist" activism—as a relevant knowledge base for discussion of fairer data arrangements. In a similar vein, we suggest investigating power struggles surrounding data infrastructures without predefined dichotomies and ideas about strong and weak partners, power and resistance, and clear-cut categories of patients and experts. Instead, we wish to draw attention to their interweaving ambiguities and temporal shifts as multiple actors build on the infrastructures set in motion by others to meet new goals.

Our own work with these topics and the material on which we build this chapter stems from years of following the evolution of data infrastructures in Danish healthcare (Hoeyer) and user involvement in digital technologies (Langstrup). To understand how patients' participation shapes and is shaped by digital health innovation, Langstrup has followed the work of governmental agencies, healthcare practitioners, and patients working to develop digital questionnaires and infrastructures for cross-sectoral and national collections of patient reported outcome data (PRO data). Langstrup has participated in meetings, workshops, and public events related to the initiative, specifically focusing on initiatives on cancer and heart disease. She has interviewed key actors involved in the initiative. Alongside this, she is also following with collaborators the so-called "looping community" of diabetes patients who, supported by online peer communities, alter technical features of their insulin treatment with unregulated technology and without formal clinical oversight. To understand the implications of governmental attempts of empowering citizens through increased data access, Hoeyer has traced the legal history, analyzed policy documents for data initiatives, and interviewed key actors working with the decision-making processes, the practical implementation of the policies, and with health professionals using the data infrastructures in their daily life. Together we have interviewed representatives for two patient organizations taking an active involvement in the development of new questionnaires to account for patient experiences, one for chronic diseases and one for cancer. In total, we have interviewed more than 100 individuals, and here present selected informants under pseudonyms and in our own translations. Our point is not to account for a particular distribution of views or experiences in what remains a non-representative sample. We detail instead the processes of infrastructuring Danish healthcare as a way of illustrating how attempts to do the right thing tend to bring about new fractures and reasons to repair.

We present the analysis in five steps, each illustrating the intertwinement of promise, ruination, and repair, and each representing a historical layer of patient politics that are built into the infrastructure: first, the historical making of a right to healthcare. Second, governmental initiatives to establish a patient right to access the data produced through care. Third, governmental ambition of empowering patients by obliging them to produce data to evaluate healthcare. Fourth, patient activism aimed at increasing self-determination with respect to the mode of care. Fifth, activism aimed at criticizing the data infrastructures in place.

2. Denmark, Data, and the Historical Layers of Power Struggles

As in the other Nordic countries, the Danish welfare state emerged gradually out of the people's movements of the nineteenth century. The workers' movement gained strength in tandem with new collaborative economic models—the so-called "andels" movement, which encouraged shared ownership of, for example, abattoirs and dairies, as well as cooperative shops. This period was also characterized by religious awakening and a strong temperance movement. As pointed out by Swedish ethnologists, the call for greater influence of the poor was accompanied with a strong emphasis on self-control (Qvarsell 1986; Frykman and Löfgren 1987). The new movements were not welcomed by established power structures. In Denmark, however, during the recession in the 1930s, a consensus gradually emerged around a more social-democratic system and the establishment of state welfare provisions—as well as a collaborative system for negotiations between unions and employers that became known as the Danish Model (Marcussen 2010). The totalitarian regimes south (Nazi Germany) and east (Soviet Union) of Denmark contributed to an evolving consensus around the benefits of more collaborative forms of governance. Many years of violent and fierce activism thus preceded the establishment of rights that today are taken for granted by both right- and left-wing politicians, such as universal access to healthcare (Lundberg et al. 2008).

Rights rarely emerge without duties: the financing of the welfare state was a problem from its inception. In 1968, a new system was introduced to ensure comprehensive taxation. Three registries for identification purposes were established to trace each individual, all dwellings, and all enterprises. As the three registries gave everyone and everything numbers and facilitated easier tracking, they quickly proved themselves useful also for purposes other than taxation. The personal identification numbers became the entry point for all public services, including social services, education, employment, and health. The welfare state in this way came to involve a particular instantiation of the well-known double meaning of surveillance: to scrutinize and to watch over. In Danish the word for surveillance (*overvågning*) is a conjunction of the word for watching over someone (*våge over*), which has clear connotations with care.

The data accumulated using the identifying numbers quickly became too ubiquitous to be manageable as paper records. Denmark embarked on a digital adventure that came to lay the foundation for contemporary data infrastructures. Already in 1976, Denmark switched from the old census model to using the digitalized central person registry (Lange 2014). From the 1980s, public-sector digitalization became a main priority and Denmark became a digital frontrunner in a number of arenas. The registries grew in number as well as purpose. Though administrative in nature, they began to be used for research (Bauer 2014). As a consequence, patients came to be spoken for in new ways as population numbers. The international journal *Science* celebrated the opportunities for research generated through the Danish registries system, describing Denmark's population as one big cohort study and "the epidemiologist's dream" (Frank 2000, 2003). Several registries were hosted originally by patient organizations, or initiated by independent clinicians. They were not part of a national plan. Only later were they transferred to governmental agencies in processes illustrating institutional responses to locally perceived data needs.

With the surge in data volumes and new data economies emerging during the 2010s, both industry and governmental agencies began to think about the data resources also as opportunities for economic growth. The old source of income—registries for taxation purposes—gradually became inscribed in new economic imaginaries: data as assets that should be exploited (see also Vezyridis and Timmons 2017; Tarkkala et al. 2018). The dominant trope during these years characterized health data as a "gold mine" (Hoeyer 2016), the argument being that new forms of income were needed if welfare were to be sustained and developed. The obligation to deliver data that should give rise to commercial gain signals a new form of social contract between citizen and state (Prainsack 2017). The social sustainability of this contract is yet to be tested. Infrastructures from the past continue to facilitate unexpected opportunities; they never cease to redefine their purposes and give rise to unexpected benefits as well as dangers.

3. Establishing a Right to Data: Promise, Ruination, and Repair

The accumulation of data has been accompanied with increasing governmental awareness of patient interests in these resources. Interest groups such as patient associations, the Danish Consumer Council, and the DanAge association (fighting against age barriers) have contributed to such awareness. Based on data from public consultations, these groups have contributed to the governmental discourses articulating promises of empowerment through enhanced data access. In 1987, patients acquired a legal right to request access to their own hospital records, and in 1988 also to electronic records from their general practitioner. In 1998, a law was passed to gather and clarify patient rights. It had the stated purpose of ensuring patients' dignity and self-determination. It is one thing to have a right, however, and quite another to have the technical options for using it. In 2003, an internet homepage was established through which citizens could access their hospital records. The name was Sundhed.dk (*sundhed* is Danish for health). Sundhed.dk is a form of national health service online, and it quickly became the main access point for patients to their data. Extensive work went into developing standards to make data from different systems available through just one interface. Over the years, sundhed.dk has expanded from computer access only to other platforms, including tablets and phones. Besides personal health records, it is also a portal providing curated information about, for example, diseases, treatment options, and waiting times at various units. From the very beginning, the platform, which is operated in collaboration between the Danish Regions, the municipalities, and the state, has worked closely with patient associations on various projects to develop and incorporate tools for patient engagement and empowerment into the platform. Furthermore, Sundhed.dk conducts user tests to explore citizen interests relying heavily on anthropological methods for including "the patient" or "citizen voice" in their digital services (methods that are used throughout the Danish health services and governmental agencies when redesigning or evaluating services).

The integration of data from multiple sources is of value also for health professionals who receive patients from other units and whose data are not available in internal systems. To ensure that no health professional uses the access to patient records for inappropriate reasons, a system of logging has followed the data integration, and through this service, patients can check who has viewed their files. On average every year, six health professionals are caught viewing health records without authorization, for example of ex-boyfriends, ex-wives, or employees. Though built as an opportunity for emergency care—access to the records of patients in need of urgent help—the data integration also came to generate these relatively rare cases of abuse. The logging system, conversely, is a form of repair, where patients acquire tools to regain control. One patient shared her story with us of finding out that her boss had looked into her medical record to cast doubt on her absence from work. She described feeling "appalled, angry, offended, nervous, and extremely psychologically affected." The logging made it possible for her to document the unauthorized viewing of her medical data.

The logging of electronic data has had various other unintended consequences involving other types of risk. Patient record audits are well-established measures of quality assurance aimed at optimizing care, but partly as a consequence of logging, patients began complaining about health professionals having looked into their records without being their treating physician. In the course of dealing with these complaints, it was revealed that the audit practice had never been authorized in the law. In 2017, a law was passed to legalize the old practice (Hartlev and Wadmann 2018). The promise of patient empowerment backfired and necessitated legal repair work.

Attempts to minimize and control physician access to patient data through systems such as logging might also have worked against other, older practices aimed at ensuring adequate treatment for each patient. In 2019, it was reported that more than 11,000 physicians had shared patient stories through a closed Facebook group. According to media reports, they did so mostly to get feedback from colleagues in a system without governmental logs (Jyllands-Posten 2019). Facebook extracts and logs information in its own way, but it is not easily accessible to patients. This case made clear that some attempts at empowering patients had contributed to the development of new patient risks—not because anybody wanted to harm patients, but because different professional groups held different ideas about how to serve patient interests. Even attempts at repair can produce new sources of ruination.

Health professionals are not the only potential source of data leakage. When patients have access, they too can decide—or be forced—to share data

124 DATAFYING THE PATIENT VOICE

(Petersson 2020). After having opened up for patients to access their own health data, Sundhed.dk learned that individuals were sharing their access codes with others. To address this and safeguard privacy, they then developed a system of authorization to enable patients to grant others access to their records. This *repair* move aimed to make citizen access to records traceable in the same way as health professionals' access. However, when in a short period all data from general practice were made available on the portal, general practitioners reported how some patients felt *forced* to share their access also with family members who wanted to assert control over their medical appointments. Young girls, for example, faced problems when using preventative services that their parents had not sanctioned. Insurance companies and employers also capitalized on the changes; where previously they had had to pay for statements from general practitioners in cases where they were entitled to information about a given health condition, now they simply asked the patient for a printout. It was clearly cheaper for the companies to do this, but crucially it also provided them with access to far more information than they otherwise would have had. Once again, patient empowerment became an unwarranted source of disempowerment. As yet another instance of repair, Sundhed.dk developed a system of "privacy marking," where patients could choose to hide certain pieces of information not only from the view of health professionals, but also from themselves (and thereby those that might force them to grant them access to it). Infrastructures are never finished; they are continuously in processes of promissory development, ruination, and repair.

Data access can also feel disempowering, even when used as intended by policy makers. Medical doctors had for long insisted on a temporal delay of laboratory results, so that patients would hear about a diagnosis from the doctors before reading it online. This was regarded as paternalistic by policy makers and by consumer activists. In the course of investigating these infrastructural changes, we met a civil servant who had been part of implementing the removal of the time delay. It transpired that she had also had personal experiences, following which she no longer saw merit in the instant sharing of the data. She had had a tissue sample sent to a pathology laboratory, and she recalled how she began shivering as she looked up the result online before speaking to her doctor:

> I could see it was a very long test result, masses of text. That was the first thing that struck me, "there's a lot here, that's not good." And then I read "malignant" and I thought, "is that good or bad, is that good or bad, is that

good or bad?"... and then I thought "shit, I've got cancer. I've got cancer"...
I started trembling all over.

She realized there was a lot in the lab results she did not understand and began contacting people she knew who might be able to translate the technical jargon. In spite of what she knew about data privacy from her work in the health services, she began to send images and printouts to people she did not personally know, asking for help with interpreting the data that she could access but not understand. She explained to Klaus how it provoked her thinking back on the small "disclaimer" she had to click before accessing the results, which informed her that she might prefer to see a doctor before reading them: "What the f*** is that? Such political 'cover-my-ass' bullshit... of course, it won't stop me when I'm already logged on to Sundhed.dk... This is not protecting my interests." She emphasizes that for data to make sense, they must be exchanged between people who know how to understand and use them. Unlike other pieces of information she had accessed in conjunction with childbirth and infant care, she said the laboratory data "were not written for me." Following the incident, she stopped trying to discern what data she could and could not use: "I have not logged on to Sundhed.dk since." This experience shows that while the promise of empowerment through data access can be fulfilled sometimes, the new opportunities it yields can also generate a sense of ruin beyond repair.

It is not only patients who face new dangers as a result of new data infrastructures. In many hospitals, health professionals have begun wearing nametags with only their first name to protect their identity. Patients can occasionally become threatening and angry, and it is important that they cannot locate the home address of the health professionals by using online tools. Despite this, the log system on Sundhed.dk provides patients with a new means of identifying the people who have treated them—and this has had unforeseen consequences. In a particularly tragic case in 2019, a doctor was killed by a former patient. The police found a printout from Sundhed.dk where the patient had used the log to identify the doctor and six other treating health professionals (Dalsgaard 2019). Patient-empowerment policies rest on the assumption that patients are in need of leverage and pursue legitimate interests aimed at improving their own health. Sometimes, however, it might be the health professionals who are in need of protection. If infrastructures solidify previous power struggles, they also create the foundation for new forms of power abuse. Every promise of empowerment risks ruination and new calls for repair.

4. Making Patients Active: Datafying Patient Voices

While the aforementioned modifications of data infrastructures revolve around data *access*, a number of recent national initiatives are aiming more explicitly at providing a national data infrastructure that supports patients to become active and continuous *contributors of data* about themselves to public health services. One initiative concerns the collection of data on patients' experiences of the effects of the treatments they receive as they engage in cross-sectoral treatment trajectories. These are PRO data and they are increasingly collected through digital questionnaires to inform clinical decision making, enable data-driven screening, and provide aggregate data for management and research. The national PRO initiative, which started in 2016, has already been praised by the Organisation for Economic Co-operation and Development as an exemplary move toward a health system that learns from "what matters to patients" (OECD Health Ministerial Meeting 2017). While other countries are also implementing PRO data as a means for more patient-centered clinical decision making and value-based management, apparently only Denmark has a national, cross-sectoral initiative, which involves both clinicians and patients throughout the process of designing the questionnaire tools and digitally supported pathways for a number of selected treatment areas (Langstrup 2019). The PRO data initiative is just one of many aimed at "patient-centeredness" and participation through technology, but it stands out for its scale and scope; the realization of the initiative's vision would mean the continuous production, collection, use, and reuse of PRO data from a large proportion of the total patient population. Major patient associations have continuously supported the initiative by helping recruit patients. Patients participate in elaborate workshops exploring how to design the questionnaires and data pathways for specific treatment areas. For these associations, an infrastructure for PRO data is a major step towards more systematic inclusion of the (individual) patient voice in clinical as well as management matters. However, for the patients who were recruited to participate in, for example, four workshops on heart rehabilitation, the very concept of PRO data was at first unclear. Furthermore, while the participating patients generally liked the idea of being asked more about their experiences and quality of life, and engaged enthusiastically in the testing of possible questionnaires, they expressed concerns regarding their own representativeness of the whole population of heart patients. They feared that the "data work" in the form of continuous registration required by patients less resourceful than themselves would exclude some from being heard and seen. Similar concerns for new inequalities produced through these participatory data infrastructures were raised among clinicians, who in parallel workshops were responsible for ensuring the clinical quality and organizational viability of the PRO infrastructure. Still the framing—individual data collected with a questionnaire and used and shared along a patient trajectory—was given. This became clear, for instance, when a patient was rebuffed as she expressed a need to get more *answers* from the clinicians she meets, rather than questions. The workshop coordinators responded that PRO is about the patient providing answers, not posing questions.

The Danish health services are also working to establish a solution that allows patients to upload their self-tracking and wearable data to the national systems, including Sundhed.dk. The commercial tech giants' success in encouraging people to use devices 24/7 and self-track their health is both in line with public promises of datafying patient experience and—in the case of the emergent commercial health data infrastructures of Google, Fitbit, and Apple—a potential threat to public infrastructures. Whether data from patients' personal devices should be uploaded onto the established public data infrastructures—and in the end health record systems—is not without contestation. The general practitioners' association has issued a policy in which it argues against a default "data-in" model for patient-reported data (Dansk Selskab for Almen Medicine 2017). Whether it is PRO data generated through the national PRO data infrastructures or data from patients' own tracking devices, the general practitioners' association opposes the sourcing of data that they have not "ordered," and which could "contaminate" the patient record. It is for these reasons that general practitioners have not been represented at most of the participatory activities involved in the national PRO data initiative. What counts as a promise of voice for some may be seen as a risk of ruination for others.

5. Discontented Patients: Patient Activism Aimed at Increased Self-Determination

Despite all these governmental attempts at engaging and empowering patients, there are people engaged in activism who believe there are better ways to do so in the age of data-intensive healthcare. As we now turn to the patients who mobilize to affect change in the healthcare services (rather than those who are mobilized by the health services), we also look towards the classic activist position of opposition. It is important to remember, however, that even for the most well known of these, such as HIV activism of the 1990s, patient mobilization has rarely focused on dismantling healthcare systems: many forms of oppositional patient activism still have increasing access to care as a central goal. Accordingly, the types of activism to which we now turn are strikingly similar to the invited participation and "empowerment" initiatives of the welfare state: they too seek to develop and repair rather than break down or sidestep existing infrastructures. And, in most cases, they are welcomed by the authorities.

One case in point which also epitomizes the particular Danish version of collaborative governance is the international patient movement known by its hashtag #wearenotwaiting. This movement was formed after a number of diabetes patients and parents of children with diabetes in the international diabetes community began independently to change their treatment devices (sensors measuring blood glucose continuously, , and insulin pumps administering insulin intravenously). Their goal in doing so was to reduce the burden on quality of life that the strict treatment and data regime of diabetes self-care can have. In online spaces such as Twitter and Facebook, these patient innovators started organizing around what became termed DIY APS (do-it-yourself artificial pancreas system) and "looping" (creating a closed loop that administers insulin automatically). These patient innovators have stirred a lot of debate and some concern in clinical diabetes communities internationally as their innovations involve unregulated alterations undertaken without formal clinical oversight and with unapproved equipment. Some authorities, such as the Food and Drug Administration in the United States (FDA 2019), have issued public concern and critique of these activities. They have been warning patients against experimenting. In some cases, we have been told, patients have been asked to sign waivers by their treating clinician or been refused treatment equipment because they were using these methods. Most patients engaged in the movement are quite explicit about their desire to collaborate not only with clinicians but also regulators and device manufacturers. Collaborations are also starting to take place. In any case, our interlocutors state that Denmark is possibly the only country in the world where a public authority responsible for the treatment of diabetes—the Steno Diabetes Center Copenhagen (SDCC) run by the Capital Region—has issued a treatment recommendation for clinicians on patients' use of DIY management technologies. The recommendation states that while clinicians cannot endorse or directly be involved in the DIY treatment, patients "must continue to receive support and care from their diabetes healthcare providers at SDCC for all other aspects of their diabetes care" (Steno Diabetes Center Copenhagen 2019).

The so-called looping community has been very enthusiastic about this, viewing it as a bold move toward recognition and collaboration. Moreover, SDCC has invited central patient innovators to public meetings, where they have presented their solutions and results for an audience of patient advocates, clinicians, and researchers. At two events that Henriette participated in, the organizers as well as participating clinicians publicly applauded the patients for their achievements, in contrast to the concerns expressed by clinicians internationally. Also, the SDCC recently offered to house "meetups" or "build parties" where experienced DIY users guide newcomers in how to alter their devices—something which in most other countries has taken place only privately. The first event took place in October 2019 and was shared on social media by clinicians and patients. The case aptly exemplifies how a participatory-minded and innovation-oriented health system seeks to enroll rather than expel activists in order to harness their efforts toward collaborative aims. While clinicians internationally have regarded this type of activism as instances of ruination, the Danish mode of collaborative governance facilitates alternative routes from promise over ruin to repair. The process involves multiple shifts in terrain as authorities acknowledge the ruination of their own treatment promises and patients become recognized as agents of repair.

There are other forms of patient activism serving as patient-initiated attempts of repair of what some patients consider governmental failure. In Denmark, two patient associations have been active in developing their own questionnaire tools aimed at data collection in research and daily care. These associations represent cancer and chronic disease patients respectively. We interviewed two women participating in this work to understand better what they wanted to achieve. The chronic disease patient, who we call Lone, first highlighted that she really valued the online access options for patient data on Sundhed.dk: "I think one good thing about this is that I as a patient can log in and see...who's been looking into my health record." She was less enthusiastic about the various attempts of gathering patient experiences through standardized questionnaires, however, and said that "There is no great love of [the standardized patient satisfaction surveys] among patients—and it's the same all over the country. It does not feel relevant. It's the system celebrating itself." Lone had decided to join some working groups to develop better questionnaires aimed at gathering patient experiences. Some of these groups were supported by the pharmaceutical industry. She wanted to ensure that doctors—or "the system"—cared about what matters to patients. To achieve this, there was a need for more systematic methods:

> I'm particularly fond of patient rated outcomes because of how systematic they are. We're not learning anything new, but it is getting collected systematically... and thereby it is given greater attention. It's usually been something the "nice nurse" could deal with on the side because of her "big heart."

As instances of what Rabeharisoa and colleagues call evidence-based activism (2014), she wanted to present patient concerns in a manner that was convincing and scientific. A cancer representative, Hanne, similarly emphasized the need for data on patient concerns to be heard in a resource-pressured system: "The way things are now, we need data [on patient experiences] because data make people listen." They were both tired of what they called "the case-story function" of patient narratives used to generate sympathy and raise money, but not to influence the mode of care. They wanted to change the priorities in the everyday procedures of the health services and in research. Lone saw data as essential to this end because: "We won't be recognized anywhere if we can't measure this in ways that are acknowledged as evidence... We've all felt ignored when things don't appear in a formalized questionnaire." They have thus begun repairing the lack of attention to patient concerns by developing additional questionnaires. These questionnaires are supposed to make authorities and clinicians listen.

There is an irony in this form of data work, however. Though both Lone and Hanne work to create questionnaires that can datafy their primary concerns and interests, the questionnaires they develop standardize patient concerns and consume the time of health professionals. Lone thus remarked:

> When I was diagnosed in the 1980s there was very limited data collection, but ample time for the clinical dialogue. There isn't anymore because you prioritize talking about data today, and you collect so much data. There's just 10 minutes for the consultation and you need to go through all the data. The clinician is obliged to focus on these things... I sometimes refuse some tests, but I know it will cost the clinic because it counts as bad quality.

Hanne also recognized that in many ways she contributed to the making of a system that by way of datafying the patient voice gave the aggregate and the arithmetical mean priority over the individual and the personal. What she wanted was to "combine all these data with the lived life, the whole person, so that you get this back and forth... I think it's going to be fantastic! It'll facilitate better treatments. I think it can give new hope." Promises, activism, and power struggles solidify in new infrastructures through which new struggles will be fought. As they are repairing the mishaps of the past, they entrench data practices that consume time and energy, and they are aware of this conundrum already at the point of system repair, but accept that no solution is without its downsides.

6. Opposing Data Infrastructures: Data Activism against the Digital Infrastructures

There are also activist groups opposing the integration of health data altogether—those that do not simply wish to repair the infrastructure, but to replace or overcome the systems described above. Various activists and commercial operators are trying to build alternative infrastructures for health data storage, such as the organization Data for Good, or the many startups claiming to do a better job of empowerment than the government authorities.

Some forms of activism also oppose datafication and data exchange. They are relatively few, but they exist. An association called the Patient Data Association (Patientdataforeningen) has been established on the initiative of general practitioners as a reaction to the political processes making data from general practice available online (Wadmann and Hoeyer 2018). They claim to be concerned for the privacy of their patients and argue that data sharing leaves the confidentiality of the doctor–patient relationship at risk. Paradoxically, they mobilize through Facebook, perhaps the digital-economy actor most associated with intensive data sourcing. The nature of ruination and repair look very different depending on which actors the activists trust. The Patient Data Association is also a relatively elitist group. In this sense, it signals a return to the oldest forms of patient activism, in that it is mostly run by a small group of doctors, who claim to speak on behalf of patients. Members of the association are well connected and use their contacts to members of parliament to pose questions to ministers and influence the public agenda. Their promise might be to destabilize the infrastructure, rather than repairing it, but the extent to which it positions itself as within or outside the existing power structure is difficult to ascertain.

A quite different data activist initiative unfolding in the Danish context is Techfestival. Debuting in 2017 and funded by the successful Danish digital entrepreneur and millionaire Thomas Madsen-Mygdal, this three-day event is organized as an international gathering for technology innovators and entrepreneurs. The festival markets itself as being in opposition to the ideologies of Silicon Valley and big tech, aiming to promote "a new agenda that anchors technology progress in society" (Thomas Madsen-Mygdal, in promotion material from the 2017 festival). The festival has attracted a large number of entrepreneurs, who have publicly lamented their own involvement in and contribution to what they now see as a digital economy turning against the initial vision of an open and democratic digital society (Bernsen 2019; see also Geiger 2020). The festival organizers have intended to mobilize the tech industry through the festival's participatory processes. These have produced both The Copenhagen Letter (https://copenhagenletter.org/) and later The Copenhagen Catalogue (www.copenhagencatalog.org) as documents for transforming the tech industry. The Letter invites people in technology industries to sign a number of principles for more responsible technological innovation, including: "tech is not above us," "progress is more than innovation," "let's build from trust," "design open to scrutiny," and "let's move from human-centered design to humanity-centered design." The Catalogue holds 150 principles "for a new direction in tech" that can be signed individually to express support. It is a form of activism aimed at challenging the digital infrastructures that Zuboff (2019) associates with surveillance capitalism. It does not only aim to repair the infrastructure; it seeks to build a new infrastructure based on other principles and values. Whereas the Patient Data Association uses private data infrastructures to challenge the public system, Techfestival challenges the private infrastructures and the ways in which large multinational companies infiltrate and take over public infrastructures and service delivery. Both types of activism are nonetheless elitist. Both are in the business not of repair, but of pointing to ruins and articulating new promises. Techfestival is supported financially by a number of both large and small technology companies as well as by the Copenhagen Municipality and the Danish Business Authorities. There are multiple positions in play within this grid, but no organization fully outside of some form of grid.

And yet, in some ways the COVID-19 pandemic provoked hitherto unseen forms of confrontational activism aimed at undermining government health policies. From the second half of 2020 onwards, an increasing number of citizens mobilized online and took to the streets protesting against a proposed law of epidemic control. These protesters also opposed data sharing and data reuse for research. The ability of collaborative governance to repair their sense of trust, which pandemic control had left in ruins, remains to be seen.

Conclusion: Promise, Ruination, and Repair

In this chapter, we have described how Danish health data infrastructures have evolved through processes of promise, ruination, and repair. We have used this case to rethink activism as it evolves within a framework of collaborative governance. Infrastructures are never finished. They always deliver both more and less than promised, and it is in the ruins of failed promises that both patients and institutions mobilize to repair. In these moments of repair, new visions and promises emerge, and through them infrastructures evolve. Promises, ruination, and repair operate in recursive circles where no step is definitely right for all stakeholders or forever. Even acts of repair will be part of creating the infrastructures through which future problems emerge. While this may sound pessimistic, we have wanted to use the Danish case to acknowledge these power struggles as also embodying forms of care. In the course of establishing a welfare state, earlier generations fought hard to turn promises of a better life into public obligations. Without a welfare state, there probably would be fewer public data mistakes—but also fewer services available to all. This does not legitimize every use of data; rather the gravity of the entitlements at stake should serve to install precaution and care when tinkering with the system. There is no perfect healthcare system, but there are systems that seek to react when unintended effects develop—or when realizing that some people experience intended effects as unfair or objectionable.

We have emphasized how promises as well as complaints about ruination and attempts of repair can come from all quarters and do not "belong" to either activists or state institutions. On closer inspection, dichotomies are not stable: what counts as inside and outside, weak and strong, constructive and destructive, patient and expert, shifts over time. Similarly, the action going into the making of infrastructures always overflows: it is morally ambiguous in its intent as well as effect.

What type of questions does this raise for scholarly work on patient activism in an age of data-intensive healthcare? Perhaps we can begin to discern with greater clarity how scholars position themselves along lines similar to those described above for the forces at play. Some scholars seek to articulate (and realize) new promises as alternatives to the existing options; others give voice to dissatisfaction and complaints about ruination; while others, again, work alongside people in their attempts of repair. All three modes of scholarly work can take sides with governmental agencies, patient activists, or other stakeholders. Some seek authenticity in their attempts to break down existing structures; others in their attempts to make them stronger, fairer, or better tuned to the needs that their research seeks to articulate. Each form of scholarly activism probably carries elements of the same inherent moral ambiguity that we described above as characterizing attempts to shape the everyday practices of the health services.

Situatedness is also geographical, social, and political. We have described a Danish case that is in some ways extreme. The Danish experience of collaborative governance provides a particular backdrop for discussions of data infrastructures. They differ in significant ways from, for example, the Chinese proclaimed communist ambition with minimal tolerance of civil activism (Lengen 2017), as well from as the deep mistrust of state initiatives in the United States where a powerful form of activism mobilizes against what it designates as "Big State" (Feingold 1995; Jasanoff 2012). While policy discourses often claim universality, all socio-political assemblages are in a certain sense unique. Scholarly work has a particular role in creating awareness of this type of situatedness.

In our analysis above, we might have emphasized the care aspect of the welfare state too much. We can be said to have placed ourselves mainly among those opting for rights to care and thereby failed to give adequate attention to the ways in which citizens might stand to lose, for example, rights of privacy. On October 17, 2019, special rapporteur on human rights for the United Nations, Philip Alston, warned welfare states against digital data integration of the type that Denmark has so radically pursued. He forcefully suggested that "as humankind moves, perhaps inexorably, towards the digital welfare future, it needs to alter course significantly and rapidly to avoid stumbling zombie-like into a digital welfare dystopia" (UN Secretary General 2019, 19). There *is* a risk that once an infrastructure is in place, it will be used by the wrong people for the wrong things (O'Doherty et al. 2016). Tupasela and colleagues (2020) have pointed to contemporary attempts to exploit Danish data infrastructures commercially as one such deviation from original promises that can endanger trust. Danish philosopher Mads Vestergaard (2019) has warned the Danish public against the emergence of a form of "digital totalitarianism" eclipsing human dignity. By emphasizing totalitarianism, Vestergaard differs from Shoshana Zuboff's (2019) famous critique of surveillance capitalism in two respects: totalitarianism aims for controlling the soul (whereas Zuboff suggests control is aimed just at behavior) and it is linked to the state (where Zuboff suggests that commercial surveillance is accepted in the United States exactly because it is not state-centered).

Though the role of the state gives rise to concern, it could—perhaps—also become a source of hope. The hope of democratic control. The surveillance opportunities of digital infrastructures alter the conditions of possibility for mobilization against those that control the data flows; every act online today leaves a trace that can also be used against you. It is therefore critical to understand how these opportunities are used, which interests they serve, and which checks and balances keep them under control. When and how data are used to watch over (*våge over*) and mobilize repair work, and when they are used to survey and control (*overvåge*) will remain empirical questions fraught with enduring moral ambiguity. Similar technologies can have very different social implications in different locales. Just like the people we study, we as scholars are caught *in medias res*—in the processes of promise, ruination, and repair. Consequently, as Foucault (1997, 232) famously suggested, "we always have something to do."

References

Adams, V. (2016), Introduction, in V. Adams (ed.) *Metrics: What Counts in Global Health* (1–17), Duke University Press.

Bauer, S. (2014), From Administrative Infrastructure to Biomedical Resource: Danish Population Registries, the "Scandinavian Laboratory," and the "Epidemiologist's Dream," *Science in Context*, 27:2, 187–213.

Bernsen, M. (2019), *Danmark Disruptet. Tro, Håb og Tech-giganter*, Gyldendal.

Bigo, D., Isin, E., and Ruppert, E. (2019), Data Politics, in D. Bigo, E. Isin, and E. Ruppert (eds) *Data Politics: Worlds, Subjects, Rights* (1–17), Routledge.

Brown, P., Morello-Frosch, R., Zavestoski, S. et al. (2011), Health Social Movements: Advancing Traditional Medical Sociology Concepts, in B. Pescosolido, J. Martin, J. McLeod, and A. Rogers (eds) *Handbook of the Sociology of Health, Illness, and Healing* (117–37), Springer.

Callon, M., Méadel, C., and Rabeharisoa, V. (2002), The Economy of Qualities, *Economy and Society*, 31:2, 194–217.

Dalsgaard, L. (2019), Mistænkt for lægedrab i Tisvilde havde flere lægers navne på en liste. *DR*. Available at: https://www.dr.dk/nyheder/indland/mistaenkt-laegedrab-i-tisvilde-havde-flere-laegers-navne-paa-en-liste.

Dansk Selskab for Almen Medicine (2017), DSAM's politik i forhold til Patientrapporterede observationer (=PRO-data). Available at: https://www.dsam.dk/flx/dsam_mener/holdninger_og_politikker/dsam-s-politik-i-forhold-til-patientrapporterede-observationer-pro-data/.

Epstein, S. (1996), *Impure Science: AIDS, Activism, and the Politics of Knowledge*, University of California Press.

Erikson, S. L. (2012), Global Health Business: The Production and Performativity of Statistics in Sierra Leone and Germany, *Medical Anthropology*, 31:4, 367–84.

Eysenbach, G. (2001), What Is E-health? *Journal of Medical Internet Research*, 3:2, e20.

FDA (United States Food and Drug Administration) (2019), https://www.fda.gov/medical-devices/safety-communications/fda-warns-people-diabetes-and-health-care-providers-against-use-devices-diabetes-management-not.

Feingold, E. (1995), The Defeat of Health Care Reform: Misplaced Mistrust in Government, *American Journal of Public Health*, 85:12, 1619–22.

Foucault M. (1997), On the Genealogy of Ethics: An Overview of Work in Progress, in P. Rabinow (ed.) *Ethics: Essential Works of Foucault 1954–1984* (Volume 1, 253–80), Penguin.

Frank, L. (2000), When an Entire Country Is a Cohort, *Science*, 287:5462, 2398–9.

Frank, L. (2003), The Epidemiologist's Dream: Denmark, *Science*, 301:5630, 163.

Frykman, J., and Löfgren, O. (1987), *Culture Builders: A Historical Anthropology of Middle-Class Life*, Rutgers University Press.

Geiger, S. (2020), Silicon Valley, Disruption, and the End of Uncertainty, *Journal of Cultural Economy*, 13:2, 169–84.

Gupta, A. (2018), The Future in Ruins: Thoughts on the Temporality of Infrastructure, in N. Anand, A. Gupta, and H. Appel (eds) *The Promise of Infrastructure* (62–79), Duke University Press.

Hartlev, M., and Wadmann, S. (2018), Sundhedsdata og kvalitetsudvikling—et retligt kludetæppe, *Juristen*, 4, 115–28.

Hoeyer, K. (2016), Denmark at a Crossroad? Intensified Data Sourcing in a Research Radical Country, in B. D. Mittelstadt and L. Floridi (eds) *The Ethics of Biomedical Big Data* (73–93), Springer.

Hogle, L. F. (2019), Accounting for Accountable Care: Value-Based Population Health Management, *Social Studies of Science*, 1–27.

Jackson, S. J. (2017), Speed, Time, Infrastructure. Temporalities of Breakdown, Maintenance, and Repair, in J. D. Wajcman (ed.) *The Sociology of Speed. Digital, Organizational, and Social Temporalities* (169–85), Oxford University Press.

Jasanoff, S. (2012), Restoring Reason, *Science and Public Reason* (1st edition, 59–77), Routledge.

Jyllands-Posten (2019), Læger udleverer patienter i stor Facebook-gruppe, *Jyllands-Posten*. Available at: https://jyllands-posten.dk/livsstil/familiesundhed/sundhed/ECE11642660/laeger-udleverer-patienter-i-stor-facebookgruppe/.

Kennedy, H. (2018), Living with Data: Aligning Data Studies and Data Activism through a Focus on Everyday Experiences of Datafication, *Krisis: Journal for Contemporary Philosophy*, 1.

Kitchin, R. (2014), *The Data Revolution: Big Data, Open Data, Data Infrastructures and Their Consequences*, Sage.

Kjær, P., and Pedersen, A. R. (2010), *Ledelse gennem patienten: nye styringsformer i sundhedsvæsenet*, Handelshøjskolens Forlag.

Lange, A. (2014), The Population and Housing Census in a Register Based Statistical System, *Statistical Journal of the IAOS*, 30, 41–5.

Langstrup, H. (2019), "Patient-reported data and the politics of meaningful data work", *Health Informatics Journal*, 25: 3, 567–76.

Larkin, B. (2013), The Politics and Poetics of Infrastructure, *Annual Review of Anthropology*, 42, 327–43.

Lehtiniemi, T., and Ruckenstein, M. (2019), The Social Imaginaries of Data Activism, *Big Data and Society*, 1–12.

Lengen, S. (2017), Beyond the Conceptual Framework of Oppression and Resistance: Creativity, Religion and the Internet in China, in S. Travagnin (ed.) *Religion and Media in China: Insights and Case Studies from the Mainland, Taiwan and Hong Kong* (19–34), Routledge.

Lundberg, O., Yngwe, M. Å., Stjärne, M. K., Björk, L., and Fritzell, J. (2008), *The Nordic Experience: Welfare States and Public Health (NEWS)*, Centre for Health Equity Studies. Available at: https://www.chess.su.se/polopoly_fs/1.54170. 1321266667!/menu/standard/file/NEWS_Rapport_080819.pdf.

Marcussen, M. (2010), *Den danske model og globaliseringen*, Samfundslitteratur.

Merry, S. E. (2016), *The Seductions of Quantification: Measuring Human Rights, Gender Violence, and Sex Trafficking*, University of Chicago Press.

Mountford, N., and Geiger, S. (2018), (Re)-Organizing the Evolving Healthcare Market: Collaborative Governance in Bureaucratic Contexts, *Academy of Management Proceedings*, 1, 14156.

Newman, J., Barnes, M., Sullivan, H., and Knops, A. (2004), Public Participation and Collaborative Governance, *Journal of Social Policy*, 33:2, 203–23.

O'Doherty, K. C., Christofides, E., Yen, J. et al. (2016), "If You Build It, They Will Come": Unintended Future Uses of Organised Health Data Collections, *BMC Medical Ethics*, 17:54, 1–16.

OECD Health Ministerial Meeting (2017), Ministerial Statement: The Next Generation of Health Reforms, *Organisation for Economic Co-operation and Development*. Available at: https://www.oecd.org/health/ministerial-statement-2017.pdf.

Olsen, L., Aisner, D., and Mcginnis, J. M. (2007), *The Learning Healthcare System: Workshop Summary*, National Academies Press.

Petersen, A., Schermuly, A. C., and Anderson, A. (2019), The Shifting Politics of Patient Activism: From Bio-sociality to Bio-digital Citizenship, *Health*, 23:4, 478–94.

Petersson, L. (2020), *Paving the Way for Transparency: How eHealth Technology Can Change Boundaries in Healthcare*, PhD thesis, University of Lund.

Pollitt, C., Harrison, S., Dowswell, G., Jerak-Zuiderent, S., and Bal, R. (2010), Performance Regimes in Health Care: Institutions, Critical Junctures and the Logic of Escalation in England and the Netherlands, *Evaluation*, 16, 13–29.

Prainsack, B. (2017), *Personalized Medicine: Empowered Patients in the 21st Century?* New York University.

Qvarsell, R. (1986), Indledning, in R. Ambjörnsson (ed.) *I Framtidens Tjänst: Ur Folkemmets Idéhistoria* (9–19), Gidlunds.

Rabeharisoa, V., Moreira, T., and Akrich, M. (2014), Evidence-Based Activism: Patients', Users' and Activists' Groups in Knowledge Society, *BioSocieties*, 9(2), 111–28.

Ruckenstein, M., and Schüll, N. D. (2017), The Datafication of Health, *Annual Review of Anthropology*, 46, 261–78.

Sheikh, A., Sood, H. S., and Bates, D. W. (2015), Leveraging Health Information Technology to Achieve the "Triple Aim" of Healthcare Reform, *Journal of the American Medical Informatics Association*, 22, 849–56.

Slack, W. V. (1997), *Cybermedicine: How Computing Empowers Doctors and Patients for Better Health Care*, Jossey-Bass.

Star, S. L., and Ruhleder, K. (1996), Steps toward an Ecology of Infrastructure: Design and Access for Large Information Spaces, *Information Systems Research*, 7:1, 111–34.

Steno Diabetes Center Copenhagen (2019), Guidelines for the Use of Unauthorized Do-It-Yourself (DIY) Medical Technologies for the Treatment of Diabetes, *Capital Region*. Available at: https://www.sdcc.dk/presse-og-nyheder/nyheder/Documents/SDCC%20guidelines%20for%20DIY%20medical%20systems-english-version-200519.pdf.

Tarkkala, H., Helén, I., and Snell, K. (2018), From Health to Wealth: The Future of Personalized Medicine in the Making, *Future*, 1–11.

Tsing, A. L. (2015), *The Mushroom at the End of the World*, Princeton University Press.

Tupasela, A., Snell, K., and Tarkkala, H. (2020), The Nordic Data Imaginary, *Big Data and Society*, 1–13.

UN Secretary General (2019), Report of the Special Rapporteur on Extreme Poverty and Human Rights, A/74/48037. Available at: https://www.ohchr.org/en/NewsEvents/Pages/DisplayNews.aspx?NewsID=25156&LangID=E.

Vestergaard, M. (2019), *Digital Totalitarisme*, Informations Forlag.

Vezyridis, P., and Timmons, S. (2017), Understanding the Care-Data Conundrum: New Information Flows for Economic Growth, *Big Data and Society*, 1–12.

Vikkelsø, S. (2010), De elektroniske patienter: Et kollektiv eksperiment med autonomi og automatik i sundhedsvæsenet, in P. Kjær and A. Reff (eds) *Ledelse gennem patienten: nye styringsformer i sundhedsvæsenet* (131–52), Handelshøjskolens Forlag.

Wadmann, S., and Hoeyer, K. (2018), Dangers of the Digital Fit: Rethinking Seamlessness and Social Sustainability in Data-Intensive Healthcare, *Big Data and Society*, 1–13.

Wadmann, S., Holm-Petersen, C., and Levay, C. (2018), "We Don't Like the Rules and Still We Keep Seeking New Ones": The Vicious Circle of Quality Control in Professional Organizations, *Journal of Professions and Organization*, 1–16.

Wehling, P., and Viehöver, W. (2014), The Virtues (and Some Perils) of Activist Participation: The Political and Epistemic Legitimacy of Patient Activism, in P. Wehling, W. Viehöver, and S. Koenen (eds), *The Public Shaping of Medical Research: Patient Associations, Health Movements and Biomedicine* (226–45), Routledge.

Wehling, P., Viehöver, W., and Koenen, S. (2014), *The Public Shaping of Medical Research: Patient Associations, Health Movements and Biomedicine*, Routledge.

Zuboff S. (2019), *The Age of Surveillance Capitalism: The Fight for a Human Future at the New Frontier of Power*, Public Affairs.

6

Initiators, Controllers, and Influencers

Enacting Patient Advocacy Roles in Cervical Cancer Screening Policy Practices

Lisa Lindén

Introduction

Recent years have seen an integration and adaptation of new screening technologies in the healthcare sector, including the human papillomavirus (HPV) test, designed for the prevention of cervical cancer. Many European countries are currently implementing a new policy—so-called "primary HPV screening"—in their national cervical cancer screening programs. This new policy challenges a long-standing, yet debated, healthcare policy-standard: the position of the Pap smear test as "the right tool for the job" in cervical cancer screening (Casper and Clarke 1998).[1] While the Pap smear is designed to identify cellular precancerous cervical lesions that might develop into cervical cancer, the HPV test is a DNA-based method that identifies sexually transmitted, oncogenic (high-risk) HPV genotypes in the body.

This chapter looks at how patient advocates have intervened in cervical cancer screening policies to promote and enact the HPV test as the new right tool for the job. It provides a case study of patient advocates as key actors in the current fabrics and monitoring of healthcare policies. It draws upon an ethnographic case study of a Swedish patients' group, called in this chapter the Gynae Cancer Group (GCG). In 2013 the GCG, together with a professor in reproductive biology, wrote a letter[2] to the National Board of Health and Welfare (NBHW) requesting an investigation into the matter of introducing an HPV-based cervical cancer screening program in Sweden—a request the board quickly agreed to. In 2015, the NBHW decided to recommend primary HPV screening, a decision that in 2017 was followed by new national clinical guidelines directing the implementation of the new policy at the regional county council level. As with other guidelines in Europe, the new Swedish

Lisa Lindén, *Initiators, Controllers, and Influencers: Enacting Patient Advocacy Roles in Cervical Cancer Screening Policy Practices* In: *Healthcare Activism: Markets, Morals, and the Collective Good.* Edited by: Susi Geiger, Oxford University Press.
© Lisa Lindén 2021. DOI: 10.1093/oso/9780198865223.003.0006

guidelines keep the Pap smear as part of the program: Pap smears are recommended as the primary method for women under thirty years old and as the follow-up method for everyone (RCC 2019). Since 2015, the GCG has concentrated parts of its advocacy on pushing for a faster implementation of primary HPV testing and a complete removal of the Pap smear from the screening program. In this chapter, I zoom in on these advocacy practices to analyze how the GCG participates and intervenes in the enactment and implementation of cervical cancer screening policies in Sweden.

In recent years, there has been a growing scholarly attention directed at patients as policy actors, such as how, through "epistemic politics" (Epstein 2016) and "knowledge mobilization" (Rabeharisoa et al. 2014a), they manage to collectively influence health policies and, more broadly, participate in the governance of health issues (Baggott et al. 2005; Löfgren et al. 2011). As part of a societal challenging of medical practitioners' authority, a redistribution of the rights and competences between patients and experts has transformed the policy arena (Rabeharisoa et al. 2014a). Today, patient representatives and patients' groups are involved in a multitude of ways in the governance of health issues and thereby participate in redefining what constitutes the common good in healthcare (Löfgren et al. 2011). Research has taken a particular interest in the institutionalization of patient participation through processes of getting "a seat at the table" (van de Bovenkamp et al. 2010; Tomes and Hoffman 2011). For example, patient representatives have become important stakeholders in the drafting of clinical guidelines. As Baggott et al. (2005, 183) argue, "jointly produced documents on practice guidelines" have come to carry "greater credibility than those drawn by the profession acting alone."

In contrast to these forms of invited patient participation, my focus is primarily on patient activism enacted through "uninvited participation" (Wehling 2012)—that is, forms of collective action where patients and patients' groups try to influence healthcare and healthcare policies through, for example, lobbying and campaigning. Drawing on science and technology studies (STS), I focus on how the GCG assembles and mobilizes scientific knowledge along with other types of knowledge—such as cancer statistics and clinical guidelines—to provide evidence in support of the HPV test as a more accurate testing method compared to the Pap smear. I attend to how the group's mobilization of evidence intervenes in policy practices and achieves change. My chapter differs from most research in the area of patient activism in that I do not focus on the use and legitimization of "experiential" knowledge (see Bloor et al. 2020). The use of patient knowledge—such as the collection of patients' stories—is a common part of the GCG's practices. However, in its advocacy around the new cervical cancer screening program, the key focus has instead been on forms of "credentialized knowledge" (Rabeharisoa et al. 2014a), like scientific and statistical knowledge. Consequently, credentialized knowledge is also the focus of this chapter.

As I detail in my analysis, the GCG's advocacy practices around the new screening program reflect different parts of the policy process: policy initiation, implementation, and change/modification, each of which requires a different role from concerned patient advocates. In making my argument, I relate to recent STS research on "evidence-based activism" (Rabeharisoa et al. 2014a) interested in the relation between current patients' groups' intervening in the fabrics of health policies and the epistemic activities that these organizations and groups utilize to bring about significant change (Akrich et al. 2014; Bloor et al. 2020). Through this focus, I describe the enactments of patient advocacy policy roles in the GCG's "practices of evidence." My chapter contributes to existing research on patient activism by showing that patients' groups' practices of evidence also allow for and enact different patient advocacy policy roles, which are constituted in, and sparked through, policy-related practices. With this focus, I ask: How does the GCG, primarily through uninvited participation, enroll credentialized knowledge to change cervical cancer screening policies, and what does this work bring about?

In what follows, I discuss social studies of the Pap smear and the HPV test to show how patients' groups and other advocacy groups have mobilized around the two technologies. Then I move to discuss the theoretical resources on evidence-based activism and policy practices I draw upon, and from there I describe the empirical research the chapter is based on. I go on to discuss my empirical findings, and show how the GCG's practices of evidence are enacting different "patient advocacy roles" through which the GCG intervenes in policy practices. Finally, I reflect upon what the case of the GCG can say about patients' groups' uninvited participation in policy practices more broadly and the relation between such forms of engagement and notions of the common good.

1. The Role of Advocacy Groups in the Enactment of Cervical Cancer Screening Policies

Since its invention in the 1940s, the Pap smear has been controversially debated because of its high rate of so-called "false negatives" (that is, the failure to identify cervical cancer tumors or precancerous cervical lesions when they are present in the body). Casper and Clarke (1998, 258) famously argue that the Pap smear has been "massaged and manipulated" to "transform it into a reasonably 'right tool for the job.'" By focusing on what they call the "construction" of "rightness," they show that the Pap smear has been made into the "right tool" through *different actors*'" claims-making strategies' (Casper and Clarke 1998, 257, emphasis in original). They highlight how women's health and patient advocacy groups, among others, have used multiple tinkering strategies to enact the Pap smear as "good enough" and have managed to position it as the gold standard for cervical cancer screening. Tinkering strategies have included, for example, attempting to automate reading of smears and pushing for regulation of laboratories (Singleton 1995, 1998; Casper and Clarke 1998).

Hogarth et al. (2012) describe how the HPV test was increasingly integrated into existing treatment protocols while failing to fundamentally unsettle the Pap smear's leading position. In 2012, the HPV test was only approved as a follow-up method, to be used after cellular abnormalities have been detected. Therefore, they argue, Pap testing was still enacted as "the right tool for the job" (Hogarth et al. 2012, 246). In a more recent publication, Hogarth et al. (2015) reflect upon the possible changes that might occur in light of the United States (US) Food and Drug Administration's (FDA) 2015 approval of Roche Diagnostics' HPV test as a sole testing method. However, they emphasize that experts disagree on a number of issues, such as the age to start HPV screening, the best triage protocol to use and the suitable screening interval (Hogarth et al. 2015, 110). They quote a collation of US advocacy groups that wrote to the FDA critiquing the approval of sole HPV screening, saying that doing so risks replacing "a safe and effective well-established screening tool and regimen that has prevented cervical cancer successfully in the U.S. with a new tool and regimen not proven to work in a large U.S. population" (Patient, Consumer, and Public Health Coalition 2014).

The US advocacy groups emphasized that HPV testing could cause overtreatment of young women who carry the virus but have little risk of developing cervical cancer (Perrone 2014). Differently from the GCG, the groups argued that using the HPV test without the Pap smear is not very useful because many young women have HPV that will disappear without treatment. Therefore, they stressed, having an HPV test without the Pap smear to check for cytological abnormalities risks scaring many women unnecessarily. Instead of sole HPV testing or, for that matter, primary HPV screening, they advocated for co-testing which combines the HPV test and the Pap smear as the initial testing method (Patient, Consumer, and Public Health Coalition 2014).

The different positions with regards to the HPV test taken by the GCG and the US advocacy groups illustrate how patients' groups mobilize *specific sets* of evidence to enact the respective technologies' "rightness." That is, advocacy groups' enactment of "rightness" of not only the Pap smear, but also the HPV test, is enacted in and through practices of evidence, and is something "partial, situated and contingent" (Casper and Clarke 1998, 257).[3]

Hogarth et al. (2012) contrast the Pap smear's promotion by women's health advocacy groups with Roche Diagnostics' intense promotion of the HPV test. Comparable to the extensive influence from pharmaceutical companies in the promotion of HPV vaccines (see Lindén 2013, 2017), the HPV test, they write, exemplifies a trend of "the increasing importance of diagnostic companies in the development and diffusion of innovative molecular diagnostics" (Hogarth et al. 2012, 246). This chapter provides a very different story that complicates Hogarth et al.'s conclusion. As I detail in my account of the GCG's practices, the group has been, and still is, a key actor in the promotion of the HPV test as the new "right tool for the job" in Sweden.

2. Patient Activism, Policy Practices, and the Translation of Knowledge into Evidence

In STS, the most famous examples of patients' groups' mobilization are patients and activists who have intervened in the production of biomedical research, such as research into HIV/AIDS (Epstein 1996) and rare genetic diseases (Callon and Rabeharisoa 2003). This research has documented the ways in which patients and activists have brought their "experiential" knowledge into the biomedical field and have managed to impact, for example, research priority policies and treatment protocols and guidelines. Research on evidence-based activism has broadened this research agenda to incorporate patients' groups' more wide-ranging epistemic activities (Rabeharisoa et al. 2014a). This perspective seeks to analyze a form of patient activism that—often through collaborations with professionals, researchers, and policy makers—mobilizes a variety of knowledge. Evidence-based activism includes, for example, the mobilization of credentialized forms of knowledge, like statistics and surveys (Akrich et al. 2014) and clinical guidelines (Bloor et al. 2020), and often engages both invited and uninvited forms of participation (Rabeharisoa et al. 2014a).

In the GCG's policy-related practices, credentialized knowledge is enacted as evidence. In using the notion of "evidence," I analyze "the selection and articulation of knowledge statements [that] aim at providing robust knowledge on how patients' and activists' conditions or situations ought to be understood and treated" (Rabeharisoa et al. 2014a, 115). To describe the GCG's practical achievement of turning knowledge into evidence, I draw from STS work attuned to analyzing material-semiotic practices of translation (Callon 2009; Law 2013). The notion of "translation" here represents the very nature of acting: "[a]cting means translating, and translating means influencing the capacities and modalities of action, since it means establishing links, connections, circulations, exchanges of properties, and original distributions" (Callon 2009, 25).

I analyze how evidence is enacted and, through that enactment, achieved in practices that establish links and connections. Through this focus, I explore how the GCG, primarily through uninvited participation, establishes heterogeneous, material-semiotic assemblages of advocates, gynecology and public health experts, data, technologies, and political claims that enact the translation of knowledge statements into evidence. Accordingly, I understand "an assemblage" as the provisional assembly of ordering humans, materials, and claims in different heterogeneous "webs of relations" (Law 2013). I especially emphasize the material and textual objects in those webs in and through which knowledge statements are materialized, mobilized, and translated into evidence. As I will show, such objects are not only technologies, like the HPV test, but can also be what I define as "evidential objects." Such objects materialize the translation of knowledge into evidence and can, for example, be maps, letters, research articles, or clinical guidelines. These objects are then mobilized by patient advocates as evidence in support of a specific cause, such as the implementation of HPV testing. Thus, while I analyze how the GCG collaborates with researchers to intervene in policy practices, I also show how its "epistemic communities" (Akrich 2010) are dependent on sets of materials, such as evidential objects. Finally, I attend to how evidence in the GCG's practices is turned into "matters of concern" (Latour 2004) where evidence is translated into policy issues through, for example, political claims about women's health.

As made clear by the research on evidence-based activism, policies are part of heterogenous assemblages. Policy practices "assemble sets of heterogeneous actors including humans and an array of technologies such as templates, checklists and guidelines" (Gill et al. 2017, 7). These sets of heterogeneous assemblages (which may include, for example, evidential objects) enact and intervene in policies in specific ways. This means that the new cervical cancer screening program is not a singular translatable policy object that can be implemented without being changed in the process. Policy practices have unintended effects and can bring about changed and unexcepted ways of

146 INITIATORS, CONTROLLERS, AND INFLUENCERS

acting and responding (Law 2013; Law and Singleton 2014; Gill et al. 2017). For example, while the letter from the GCG to the NBHW—as an example of uninvited participation—played a crucial role in the enactment of a primary HPV screening policy in Sweden, not all the requests from the GCG have, so far, been translated into actual clinical practices, and changes have occurred along the way. Some of these changes are in line with the GCG's requests in its letter to the NBHW, while others are not. However, all of them have sparked new actions and responses from the GCG. Thus, as I detail in my analysis, changes and unintended effects can spark new policy issues which can then prompt new patient advocacy actions in response. As I will show, this allows for an understanding of patient advocacy policy roles as collective achievements that are enacted in and through heterogeneous assemblages and in relation to responses to previous advocacy and/or policy actions and requests.

3. Healthcare Context, the Study, and Its Methods

This chapter draws upon an ethnographic project exploring the practices of gynecological cancer patients' groups and is based on fieldwork between April 2018 and September 2019, as well as analysis of documents and online data. The project has been granted ethics approval, and names of participants and the organization have been anonymized. The empirical material consists of twenty-one observations of board and working group meetings in-person and online (the GCG holds both forms of meetings), as well as observations of six seminars, two patient webinars, and two patient council meetings. The seminars were directed at patients, practitioners, and scientists with the joint purpose of providing knowledge and advocating for change. The data also include sixteen in-depth interviews with GCG board members, ex-board members, and volunteers.[4]

Online material from the organization's webpage and social media channels, as well as documents such as newsletters and opinion articles written by members of the organization, are part of the dataset. This additional material is comprised of: the letter the GCG sent to the NBHW in 2013 and the subsequent correspondence between the organizations; all status updates from the GCG's Facebook site about the new screening program (in total eighty-three status updates, from 2015 to 2019); two opinion articles about the new screening program written by the GCG and published in local newspapers; and four print and television interviews with GCG representatives about the program.

In Sweden, patient associations are commonly funded by the state, but such funding is conditioned on associations utilizing a structure of national alliance with local chapters. As the GCG operates as a group without local chapters, it stands outside such funding (the GCG representatives explain this decision as resulting from their desire to focus on their "causes" instead of "getting stuck" in bureaucracy). The organization's board members and volunteers have personal experience of cancer or cancer risk (e.g. cytological abnormalities) and/or are relatives of cancer patients. The group consists of people in their twenties to senior citizens, and all are women. The majority work part or full time in another profession and participate in the GCG during evenings and weekends. The organization is focused on increasing the public's and professionals' knowledge about gynecological cancers, influencing healthcare and research, and providing support to women affected by gynecological cancers and their relatives. Advocacy surrounding the new screening program is one important part of its work, but other major areas include campaigns aimed at increasing women's knowledge about ovarian cancer, pushing for increased ovarian cancer research funding, and managing its online support groups. During my fieldwork, the group consisted of eight to twelve board members and working groups of four to six members (including board members and sometimes additional people). The organization was founded in 2007, has approximately 1,300 members, and has no paid staff.

The cervical cancer screening program was introduced in Sweden in the 1960s and is offered to all Swedish women aged 23–64 years. Since its introduction, cervical cancer has gone from being the third largest cancer amongst Swedish women to become the seventeenth. The decrease in the prevalence of cervical cancer in Sweden is equivalent to that seen in other countries with national screening programs (RCC 2019).

4. The GCG's Cervical Cancer Screening Policy Advocacy Practices

Here I describe the GCG's practices of intervening in cervical cancer screening policies in Sweden. I analyze its practices and "causes" of (1) initiating the new primary HPV screening policy; (2) speeding up the implementation of the screening policy; and (3) removing the Pap smear from the policy. In my analysis I show how each "cause" enacts a specific policy role for the GCG advocates that directs how they act and what knowledge they translate into evidence.

148 INITIATORS, CONTROLLERS, AND INFLUENCERS

4.1 Initiating the New Cervical Cancer Screening Policy: "Saving Women's Lives"

> Cytology has a sensitivity of approximately 70% and it decreases with a woman's age... HPV can be detected with very sensitive methods, with a sensitivity that is not far from 100%... Just recently, a study was published in *The Lancet*, in which it was shown that screening based on HPV gives a 60 to 70% better protection against the development of cervical cancer than screening based on cytology does... We want... a speedy transition from cytology-based screening to HPV-based screening. (Excerpt from Letter to the NBHW, 2013)

In the letter to the NBHW, the GCG, together with a professor in reproductive biology, emphasized that HPV testing is a more sensitive method compared to cytology, that is, the Pap smear. "Sensitivity" is a "probability of detection" metric that measures the proportion of so-called actual positives and is commonly used to determine the relative value of screening technologies (Armstrong and Eborall 2012). In this context, sensitivity measures the percentage of women who are correctly identified as being, in the case of the HPV test, high-risk HPV-positive, and in the case of the Pap smear, as having cytological abnormalities. By emphasizing the Pap smear's lower sensitivity in its letter, the GCG mobilized what Casper and Clarke (1998, 263) define as the Pap smear's "chronic ambiguities," such as difficulties in reading the screening slides and placing them into the cervical cancer classification systems. In the letter, the statistical knowledge produced via the sensitivity metric, as a form of credentialized knowledge, was translated into evidence for why the HPV test is the new "right tool" for the cervical cancer screening program. This was done through establishing a link between the sensitivity metric and a specific solution: "a speedy transition" to HPV-based screening.

When I met with GCG board member Karin for an interview, she referred to the article in *The Lancet* (Ronco et al. 2010) mentioned in the letter as important for its decision to write to the NBHW. Karin said that the article, which reports results from a randomized controlled trial of HPV-based versus cytology-based screening, shows that the HPV test is a better test than the Pap smear. Karin explained that she brought up the article when she talked with a scientist specializing in cervical cancer screening during a seminar. In mobilizing the article from *The Lancet* as evidence—what I call an "evidential object" for a possible need to change the screening method in Sweden—she asked the scientist why Sweden did not use the HPV test as the primary testing method. The researcher, Karin told me, answered that Sweden was in no hurry to change its method, as such a change would not affect that many women or save that many women's lives. This made Karin angry:

> I got so angry! I thought, like, how can you talk about women's lives in that way?...It turned out then that we talk about 30 [saved] lives a year and 60 [less] people diagnosed yearly. [A healthcare practitioner] sat pretty much behind me and then I said to her, you know, "what to do?" and she said "but send a letter to the NBHW"...[The professor] joined, so he and I wrote a letter. (Karin)

While both Karin and the researcher agreed that "women's lives" was an important matter, it seems, based on Karin's account, that they came to different conclusions. The researcher probably drew upon population health data to enact the number of women's lives saved to be too small, but Karin enacted a different "politics of numbers" (Rabeharisoa et al. 2014b) in which small numbers of saved lives also matter.

During my fieldwork, the GCG representatives frequently emphasized that gynecological cancers are not prioritized as they concern women's health and sex organs. For example, GCG board member Alzena said in one interview that "gynaecological cancer is an under-prioritized area" and in another interview said: "People don't want to talk about those things that afflict women." Similarly, GCG board member Mia said: "[I]t's about, you know, sex organs, purely female organs and I don't think it's interesting enough for the professionals." Karin herself emphasized that gynecological cancers are not frequently talked about and are not that well known because they are connected to women's sex organs. Against this backdrop, it's easy to understand why Karin would say "I got so angry!" and "how can you talk about women's lives in that way?" because she felt that the researcher talked about women's lives as not being important enough.[5] However, this political claim about an underprioritization of women's health was not included in the GCG's letter to the NBHW. Instead, the letter focused on scientific and statistical evidence. As I will show, this partly differs from other parts of its practices.

Karin explained to me that she teamed up with the professor she co-wrote the letter with because his viewpoints were in line with the GCG's. This is common for how the GCG works to change healthcare policies. As Karin said in an interview: "We chose people who have the same opinions as we do." As is common for current patients' groups (Panofsky 2011; Rabeharisoa et al. 2014a), the GCG representatives keeps themselves updated on recent

150 INITIATORS, CONTROLLERS, AND INFLUENCERS

developments in the field and push for the introduction of new treatments and technologies they consider would benefit their patients' group. Like Karin did in the encounter described above, the GCG participates in seminars (and conferences) and its members socialize with researchers, policy makers, and practitioners in such settings. Through these activities the GCG has built an "epistemic community" (Akrich 2010) of likeminded experts, and these experts help the GCG select and strengthen its credentialized knowledge. Based on his research on HPV testing, the reproductive biology professor who co-authored the letter has long argued for the HPV test as more accurate and efficient when compared to the Pap smear and was thus a fitting collaborator.

Through the collaboration with the professor and writing the letter, the GCG enacted a form of patient activism that can be defined as being "initiators": to put a new issue on the policy agenda. Importantly, the letter to the NBHW, *The Lancet* article, the sensitivity metric, the professor, and the GCG together enabled and enacted this patient advocacy role. It was a collective achievement; the GCG needed these heterogeneous elements to, via uninvited participation, initiate the policy change. As a key actor in this heterogeneous assemblage, the GCG collected biomedical and statistical knowledge in support of its cause and made an alliance with the reproductive biology scientist.

While the US advocacy groups mentioned by Hogarth et al. (2015) argued for the continued importance of the Pap smear, knowledge in support of the Pap smear was left out of the assemblage gathered by the GCG. This exclusion is not a surprise, but it highlights that the GCG assembled a *specific* set of knowledge and expertise. The letter to the NBHW was here a key element, as it enabled the GCG to enact the cervical cancer screening program as a public health issue in need of policy attention and to translate its selected scientific and statistical knowledge into evidence supporting the superiority of the HPV test over the Pap smear. As I will show, when the letter was translated into clinical guidelines and, later on, into clinical practice, changes occurred that also sparked new advocacy actions from the GCG and new roles in the process.

4.2 Speeding Up the Implementation of the New Screening Policy: "It's Unequal Healthcare"

In its letter to the NBHW, the GCG requested "a speedy transition" to HPV-based screening. Since several county councils have not yet fully implemented the new screening program, the GCG currently works intensely to speed up this process. In this section I will attend to how the GCG mobilizes evidence to enact the message that, as the group frequently writes on its Facebook site, "HPV testing needs to be implemented NOW." I will show that the very fact that the GCG's request for a "speedy transition" has, in many county councils, not been translated into clinical practice is important to understanding this advocacy practice.

Every year the GCG organizes gynecological seminars in about four cities for, and with, healthcare practitioners, scientists, and concerned members of the public. During a presentation of the GCG's focus and viewpoints at a 2019 seminar, Karin stressed how the GCG found the slow pace of implementation to be problematic. I wrote the following fieldnote:

> Karin highlights that the new cervical cancer screening guidelines were already ready in 2017 and that the county councils have had since 2015 to prepare for the new HPV screening program. On the PowerPoint, she presents a map of Sweden from the NBHW showing that only a total of 9 out of 20 county councils have implemented the new program. "It's awful, we think," she says. She sounds concerned and continues: "We are ashamed of all you county councils who have not yet implemented the new screening program." "You don't care about your women," she emphasizes. She states that many women would get to live if the new program would be implemented right away. "It would save lives," she says forcefully. On the PowerPoint it is written: "A big failure." (Fieldnotes, April 4, 2019)

Karin used the presentation as an opportunity to push concerned actors to take action to make sure that the screening program would be in place as soon as possible. In her presentation, the guidelines directing the implementation were enacted as evidence supporting the view that the current situation was "a big failure" ("the new guidelines were already ready in 2017," as she said), and the guidelines, as a form of credentialized knowledge, were mobilized to speed up the process. By stressing that "it's terrible" and "a big failure," the slow implementation process was enacted as a "matter of concern" (Latour 2004). The fact that the new guidelines had not yet been translated into clinical practice in several counties—the implementation process could be considered as not speedy—enables this advocacy practice devoted to speeding up the implementation process. Hence, it is the very *lack of* action from concerned county councils that has sparked this patient activism. I will return to this.

Karin's presentation enacted the uneven implementation of the new policy as a case of unequal healthcare: some women are protected by the HPV test and others are stuck with the less good Pap smear. As is shown in the excerpt above, she used a map in the presentation that had originally been produced by the NBHW to visualize the implementation process. Together with the guidelines, the map was translated into evidence for the message that the slow implementation of the program was a case of unequal healthcare. Moreover, the map enabled Karin to translate their case of unequal healthcare into a political issue about underprioritization of women's health: "you don't care about your women," as she said in the presentation.

During my fieldwork, the map from the NBHW has frequently been enrolled by the GCG as evidence for its case that the uneven implementation process amounted to unequal healthcare. The map can be understood as credentialized knowledge: it is a map used and designed by the NBHW to represent the current situation concerning the implementation process. Moreover, the map is an "evidential object" that materializes the GCG's claim that the implementation process is a case of unequal healthcare. For example, the group has frequently posted the latest version of the map on its Facebook page followed by the message that the implementation "needs to happen NOW." Similarly, the map was presented by Karin at a board meeting in August 2019 to some of the new board members as "all we really need to know." She emphasized that the map shows which county councils their efforts need to target, i.e. the county councils that have not yet implemented the new program. With an agitated tone she said that it was "god damn indefensible" that several county councils still hadn't implemented the guidelines. During situations like these, the map has enabled the GCG to translate the implementation process into a matter of unequal healthcare and into evidence supporting this claim.

In this practice, unequal healthcare is a matter of not following the new national guidelines for the screening program. This was, for example, made clear during the board meeting discussed above. At the meeting the board linked "not following the guidelines" to "unequal healthcare," as is illustrated in this excerpt from my fieldnotes:

> The group talks about the county councils that have not yet implemented the new screening program. The board member Marie emphasizes that it is problematic with "regional differences" and that it should be "equal." She stresses that it should not have to be that you live in "the right" county council to get the recommended treatment. Karin responds: "That's how it is, [healthcare in] Sweden is not equally distributed." She emphasizes that there needs to be a "joint lowest level." In relation to a later discussion during the

meeting about a county council that is not following the ovarian cancer guidelines concerning the use of the cancer antigen blood test CA125, Maria refers back to her previous comment and says that this is what she means with equal healthcare. She argues that the guidelines need to be the "joint lowest level." Karin nods and says, rhetorically: "What are the guidelines worth if some [county councils] override them?"

(Fieldnotes, August 31, 2019)

As described in my fieldnotes, the board members and volunteers at the meeting came to a joint understanding of unequal healthcare being a matter of not following the guidelines. In defining "the guidelines" as the "joint lowest level," county councils not following them are, therefore, contributing to unequal healthcare. This directs how the GCG understands its role in relation to the county councils that have yet not implemented the new program. Here, the group's role becomes a matter of making sure that the county councils "do what they should." Thus its role becomes holding the county councils accountable for their *lack of* action and pushing them to act. This is also how it is possible to understand Karin's presentation at the seminar described above, where she mobilized the map as evidence for the implementation being slow. The presentation was pushing concerned county councils to act. In this practice, the translation of the guidelines into evidence for the implementation process as a matter of unequal healthcare is crucial. As with the map previously discussed, the guidelines as a credentialized "evidential object" helps enact the implementation process as a matter of concern; the fact that the guidelines have existed since 2017 enables the message that the process is slow.

This is a patient advocacy practice that has to do with what the volunteer Malena described in an interview as being "controllers." This can be understood as a form of patient activism that holds concerned healthcare institutions accountable by "controlling" whether they follow regulations or recommendations and, if they don't, pushes them to do so. Differently from the role as initiators, the role as controllers aligns with the implementation part of the policy process and is, for example, devoted to making the translation from clinical guidelines to clinical practice happen. This form of activism in the GCG's practices is enabled by the enactment of the implementation process as "slow" and "a failure" and can be understood as an unintended effect of the letter to the NBHW. That is, the fact that the GCG's request for a "speedy transition" has not been translated into clinical practice in several counties has given rise to this new advocacy role.

Mobilizing around the slow implementation process as a matter of unequal healthcare is one way of acting as controllers. In recent years, the GCG has frequently emphasized in the media that several county councils have not implemented the new screening program. For example, in December 2018, the board member Mia was interviewed in the media.[6] In the interview she stressed that it is "disrespectful" that several county councils do not follow the guidelines, and she said that she sometimes "wonders if it's less prioritized because it concerns women's health." Similarly, in September 2019 the media reported that many county councils do not follow the cervical cancer screening guidelines. One of the key messages was that of unequal healthcare between the regions. As a response to this, the GCG wrote on its Facebook page that "it's a full-blown healthcare scandal" that several county councils have not implemented the new program. Commenting on an article where the Swedish Cancer Society directed strong critique towards these county councils, it thanked the organization "for supporting Swedish women in this question." As these examples illustrate, in the GCG's practices of speeding up the implementation process, unequal healthcare is enacted as a matter of concern that makes women's lives and health in general, and by some regions in particular, underprioritized. In this practice of mobilization as "controllers," its evidence for the implementation being slow is translated into a political claim about an underprioritization of women's health. It also allows it to enact itself as "controller" holding concerned county councils accountable for this very issue: the turning of the implementation of the new cervical cancer screening policy in Sweden into a matter of unequal healthcare.[7]

4.3 Pushing for Sole HPV Screening: "The Quality of the Pap Smear Is Extremely Bad"

When the GCG received the answer from the NBHW that a possible introduction of a new screening program would be reviewed, the group reported enthusiastically about this via its online channels. However, it also underlined that it would "try to influence those things we believe can be even better." In this section, I will attend to two core matters the GCG takes issue with in the new policy guidelines: the continued use of the Pap smear for women under thirty and the use of it as the follow-up method for all ages.[8] The GCG mobilizes evidence for a policy that recommends an HPV-positive result be followed up with a renewed HPV test after six to twelve months and that if the result is still positive, the woman should be referred for a colposcopy. In the current guidelines, colposcopy is used, if needed, after follow-ups with the Pap smear. The GCG's position can be compared to that being adopted in Australia, where women are referred directly to colposcopy if the HPV test comes back positive (Cancer Council Australia 2017). The GCG responded to the NBHW, and wrote:

> The NBHW's proposal to introduce the HPV test at age 30 is too late. We believe that the HPV test should be introduced at age 25, as the number of new [cervical] cancer cases in Sweden is almost as many for women aged 25 to 29 years old as for women aged 30 to 34. This indicates that there already today are problems with the Pap smear, and that [it] should be replaced with a more sensitive test... Furthermore, we are concerned that the follow-up of HPV-positive women with cytology is not a sufficiently sensitive method for women over 30 year of age... We are aware of existing research reports on how cytology as a follow-up method, following an HPV-positive test, reduces the risk of cancer, but these are not enough. One can clearly see in the NBHW's statistics that the number of new cancer cases is highest for women between 30 and 59 years old. For this age group, the screening program should provide an adequate follow-up procedure with a sensitive test as the HPV test, not a less sensitive test such as the Pap smear.
>
> (Excerpt from Response to the NBHW, 2014)

The new clinical guidelines do not recommend HPV testing for women aged twenty-five–thirty because "there is no scientific support for the HPV testing being a more effective testing method than Pap testing for this age group" (RCC 2019, 19). The NBHW writes that there is a risk for overtreatment if the HPV test is used for this age group (RCC 2019, 19), a position that is also held by the advocacy groups mentioned in Hogarth et al. (2015). Moreover, it is emphasized that the use of the Pap smear as the follow-up method is based on scientific evidence showing that this combination provides a sensitivity of 100 percent for the detection of persistent severe cytological abnormalities (RCC 2019, 96–7). However, the GCG had already contested these claims in 2014. As is shown in its response to the NBHW excerpted above, the high rate of cervical cancer in younger ages, as well as the even higher rate for women aged thirty–fifty-nine, was used by the GCG to problematize research on the continued relevance of the Pap smear. Hence, the GCG intervened in the fabrics of the cervical cancer screening policy through a critical engagement with the scientific and statistical state-ments enacted in the NBHW's suggestion for new clinical guidelines. Here,

156 INITIATORS, CONTROLLERS, AND INFLUENCERS

statistics is an especially important credentialized form of knowledge the GCG uses to intervene in policy.

As the NBHW has not adhered to the GCG's suggestion to fully remove the Pap smear from the guidelines, the GCG currently engages in a form of activism devoted to pushing for its removal. In an interview, Karin explained to me that the GCG does not understand why the NBHW holds on to the Pap smear in its guidelines. "The quality of the Pap smear is extremely bad," she emphasized. "Why should you use cytology to double-check? For that, [the] HPV [test] is much better and safer. We didn't understand that, [and] we still don't understand that." This was also raised by Karin during a board meeting in August 2019: "One better test is controlled by a less good test. Why? Something went wrong in their thinking there." These empirical examples provide an important backdrop for the GCG's current advocacy practice of pushing for the removal of the Pap smear.

Differently from its role as initiator and controller, the GCG intervenes as policy "influencer" in its advocacy pushing for the removal of the Pap smear. Whereas the "controller" tries to make sure that concerned actors, such as policy implementers, do what it has been decided they should do, the "influencer" pushes for further policy changes. Through its role as influencer, the GCG mobilizes to "influenc[e] the capacities and modalities of action" (Callon 2009, 25) by assembling sets of evidence together enacting support for further changes in the new policy. Importantly, the tension between the GCG's request in 2013 for sole HPV testing and the NBHW's decision to keep the Pap smear as the follow-up method has enabled this role of being influencer and sparked this activism. Hence, as with its role as "controller," its role as "influencer" can be understood as being sparked by *the response from* concerned credentialized experts to the group's requests.

In its role as influencer, the sole HPV testing policy adopted in Australia is translated into evidence for the need to also adopt a similar policy in Sweden. For example, at the above-mentioned board meeting, the group referred to how it was reported in the fall of 2018 that "Australia is close to eradicating cervical cancer" (e.g. Omni 2018) thanks to its policy. At another meeting, Karin said rhetorically: "Why should we be less good than they are in Australia?"

During the fall of 2018, the GCG mobilized the news about Australia in its practices, which serves as a good example of how it acts as influencer, through uninvited participation. In a post on Facebook, the GCG shared a media interview with a scientist. The scientist stressed that Australia was close to eradicating cervical cancer after an HPV-based screening program as well as

HPV vaccination campaign for both boys and girls had been introduced there. Commenting on this, the GCG emphasized that all women in Sweden need to be offered the HPV test as they are in Australia. Hence, the interview with the scientist, as well as the Australian guidelines, were translated into evidence in support of the need for Sweden to use HPV testing for younger girls as well as the follow-up method for positive HPV test results. Thus, the existence of the "HPV test friendly" Australian guidelines enabled the GCG to both translate the NBHW's refusal to introduce a sole HPV testing program in Sweden into a matter of concern and to act as influencer pushing for further change in the new Swedish policy. Here, the Australian guidelines can be understood as a credentialized "evidential object" making the translation of knowledge into evidence possible.

The Swedish media also reported in 2018 that cervical cancer was increasing in the group of women who have received a negative Pap smear result, i.e. among women that received a letter stating that they don't have cytological abnormalities (Swedish Cancer Society 2018). A report conducted by representatives from the Swedish Cancer Registry indicated that some laboratories have particularly high rates of false negatives, and the report argued that this seemed to be one of the reasons for the increased cervical cancer rates (Dillner et al. 2018). In evoking some of the Pap smear's "chronic ambiguities" (Casper and Clarke 1998, 263), the report seemed to imply that cytotechnicians at specific laboratories too often misread the Pap slides, and/or assign slides a classification degree not in accordance with reality. The investigating team emphasized that concerned county councils need to implement the new primary HPV screening program as soon as possible (Dillner et al. 2018).

The GCG mobilized the media coverage about the wrong test results as evidence for the need to remove the Pap smear from the program. In one news report, a journalist explained that the problem resulted from "the human factor." When commenting on this in a media interview, Karin stressed that the GCG wants "a mechanical analysis of the test, that is, an HPV analysis." On its Facebook page, the GCG shared the link to the media interview with Karin and wrote: "HPV analysis of the tests is one of our demands. Another cytotechnician that has made a mistake! HPV analysis is mechanical and a much better analysis method." Hence, the HPV test as a "mechanical method" was promoted by problematizing the manual readings of the Pap screening slides. Such problematizations of the quality of the laboratories have, seemingly paradoxically, facilitated the durability of the Pap policy-standard in previously Pap-based policies (Casper and Clarke 1998; Singleton 1998). In contrast, in the GCG's practices, they are translated into evidence for why the

158 INITIATORS, CONTROLLERS, AND INFLUENCERS

Pap smear *itself* is the problem. This mobilization of media as evidence plays a role in enacting the GCG's role as policy influencer. While media, in itself, is not always considered to be credentialized knowledge, the selection of media coverage the GCG assembled and mobilized was focused on such knowledge.

The GCG did not mobilize media coverage positive towards the continued existence of the Pap smear. This is not surprising but further highlights that the GCG, as in its initial letter to the NBHW, assembled *specific* knowledge. In response to the report from the Swedish Cancer Registry, the professional organization *Sveriges Cytodiagnostiker* (Cytodiagnostics in Sweden) wrote an opinion article where it emphasized that it is wrong to blame a whole professional group for the increase in cervical cancer cases (Dahl-Olausson et al. 2019). The organization problematized that primary HPV screening was presented as the most pressing solution and asked for support in improving the quality of cytology. It emphasized that sometimes the Pap slides show cytological abnormalities (of the classification kind "high grade squamous intraepithelial lesion") while the HPV analysis is negative. Similar to the advocacy groups in Hogarth et al. (2015), it emphasized that it therefore is problematic to assume that no cytological abnormalities exist if the HPV test is negative. Consequently, it stressed that the Pap smear is needed as a follow-up method (Dahl-Olausson et al. 2019). Similarly, one scientist wrote on the GCG's Facebook page in the fall of 2018 emphasizing that the Pap smear is needed as a follow-up method and that efforts should therefore be focused on improving the quality of cytology. A couple of weeks later he wrote again, suggesting the GCG "collaborate/discuss also with the cytology side." Karin responded to the first message, emphasizing that the choice of method is purely "based on evidence," but neither she nor any other GCG member responded to the second post. The GCG's exclusion of cytology expertise—including arguments made by "the cytology side" for the need to keep the Pap smear as the follow-up method— facilitates its advocacy for removing the Pap smear from the guidelines and is understandable considering its "cause" of mobilizing for sole HPV screening. However, the position taken by the US advocacy groups mentioned by Hogarth et al. (2015) elucidates that it could have been otherwise; an advocacy practice more in line with "the cytology side" could have been possible.[9]

Conclusion

In this chapter I have described how the GCG engages in "evidence-based activism" (Rabeharisoa et al. 2014a) in its practices of mobilizing for the HPV test as the new "right tool for the job" (Casper and Clarke 1998) in Swedish cervical cancer screening. The chapter provides a case study of how patient activism via uninvited participation (Wehling 2012) can facilitate the unsettling of long-standing policy-standards—in this case, the Pap smear—in healthcare practice. As such it also problematizes Hogarth et al.'s (2012) conclusion that the HPV test exemplifies a new trend where diagnostic companies rather than advocacy groups—such as patients' groups—push for the diffusion and adoption of new molecular diagnostics. In contrast to this conclusion, the case of the GCG exemplifies how patients' groups today are key actors in the fabric and monitoring of policies in the healthcare complex, and how they, through collective action outside of invited forms of participation at the policy table, can achieve significant change.

I have argued that the GCG's advocacy practices include the enactment of specific patient advocacy roles: "initiators," "controllers," and "influencers." My chapter provides insights on how such roles are dependent on advocates, professionals, materials, and political claims, which enact them in and through specific practices. Understood in this way, patient advocacy policy roles are collective, material-semiotic achievements. I have especially emphasized what I have defined as "evidential objects." By conceptualizing objects such as maps, guidelines, and research articles, that materialize patients' groups' translation of knowledge into evidence as "evidential objects," I argue that it is possible to further understand the role of material and textual objects in evidence-based activism. Such objects seem to be crucial for patients' groups' knowledge-related advocacy practices (Akrich et al. 2014; Rabeharisoa et al. 2014a, 2014b; Bloor et al. 2020), and my study specifically suggests that they participate in constituting different patient advocacy roles. They take part in directing how patients' groups act and what evidence they mobilize in doing so.

The chapter suggests that we understand patient advocacy roles as enacted and constituted in relation to other actors'—such as policy makers and policy implementers—responses to patient advocates' requests. In the case of the GCG, the advocacy roles as controller and influencer were enabled by the unintended effects occurring when its policy requests were, or were not, translated into clinical guidelines and clinical practice. That is, how policy makers and policy implementers *responded to* the GCG's claims and requests was also what sparked new action from the group and enacted its roles as controller and influencer. This shows that patients' groups' actions can productively be understood as "relational effects" enacted as responses to other actors' responses. Seen in this way, patient activism is a dynamic relational response to public and political issues enacted in and through health (policy)

160 INITIATORS, CONTROLLERS, AND INFLUENCERS

practices. This attention to the collective achievement of advocacy roles and actions is important to further understand the dynamics of patient activism, i.e. how it is enabled, sparked, and achieved.

In the introduction I wrote that patients and patients' groups participate in redefining and constituting "the common good" in healthcare. Let's now, finally, return to this. The mobilization of evidence responding to a policy issue is how the GCG mobilizes for and enacts the common good in healthcare. Unlike, for example, the early breast cancer (Klawiter 2008) and childbirth (Akrich et al. 2014) feminist movements, it would be difficult to relate this patient activism to a specific ideology. Instead it mobilizes around "knowledge" and enacts the common good through "a politics of numbers" (Rabeharisoa et al. 2014b) that pays close attention to the individual person or patient. This suggests that understanding current forms of patient activism requires more than analyzing what specific ideologies patient advocates draw upon to describe themselves and to mobilize for the common good. Instead, my chapter highlights how the common good is dependent on material-semiotic assemblages that diverse actors, including patients' groups, engage with. The common good is then enacted in and through practices, rather than being an abstract construction based on general ethical or political principles. Therefore, it seems essential to further attend to the heterogeneous assemblages through which different versions of the common good—and different roles and collective actions—are realized and achieved in patients' groups' practices of evidence.

Acknowledgments

The chapter has benefited greatly from comments from two anonymous reviewers and the editor of this volume, as well as from Choon-Key Chekar, Maria Eidenskog, Doris Lydahl, Anna Mann, and Vicky Singleton. It is part of my research project "Empowerment and Stigmatization: Patient Organizations, Gynecological Cancer and Changing Identities," funded by the Swedish Research Council (VR-2017-00243).

Notes

1. Certain strains of HPV might develop to cervical cancer, but the majority of HPV infections spontaneously resolve within two years (NCI 2019; RCC 2019).
2. The letter is on the GCG's home page. The reference is not included here due to anonymity reasons.

3. The US guidelines recommend any of the three methods (Pap, HPV, or co-testing) (NCI 2019). The policy differences between Europe, the US, and, as I will discuss, Australia well illustrate that the "rightness" of both the Pap smear and the HPV test is partial and contested.

4. All data are translated from Swedish into English by the author.

5. The GCG's enactment of gynecological cancer as underprioritized can be contrasted with the vast public attention to and fundraising for breast cancer (see Chapter 7 in this volume). The early breast cancer movement was essential in the turning of breast cancer into a public issue; it forcefully pushed for more research, better treatments, and higher public visibility (Klawiter 2008).

6. In the interview, Mia's own cervical cancer experience was included. She explained that during her cervical cancer treatment, she realized that the healthcare system did not work too well, and she decided to get involved in the GCG to do something about it. This is one of the few examples I have seen where patient experience—or "experiential knowledge"—has been mobilized as evidence in the GCG's practices around the new cervical cancer screening program.

7. The new screening program requires a new information technology system, and unclear orders from the county councils concerning this have been highlighted as one key reason for why not all county councils have implemented the new screening program (Swedish Cancer Society 2018). To speed up the delivery of the new system, the GCG has been in contact with the concerned system company and has connected it with a key policy maker in the context of the new screening program via a conference call. This can be compared with Panofsky (2011), who describes how patients' groups try to influence the direction of, in his case, biomedical research, by acting as a "facilitator" that establishes contact between key actors in the medical field.

8. The GCG also pushes for older women's access to the HPV test as well as for the possibility to do a "HPV self-test" at home, but this is outside the scope of this chapter.

9. It is worth reflecting upon how quickly the NBHW after the GCG's suggestion adopted the new "primary HPV screening" policy and, thus, how quickly the GCG managed to achieve significant policy change. Part of this likely has to do with the timing of the GCG's suggestion; other European countries started initiating HPV-based screening around the same time. Still, looking more broadly, during my fieldwork I have noticed the relative lack of apparent resistance towards the GCG by credentialized experts. The group has during latter years managed to gather not only an "epistemic community" of like-minded experts, but also, more generally, to gain a position in Swedish gynecological cancer healthcare as a stakeholder with significant expertise and credibility. Nevertheless, in interviews I have conducted, the GCG participants have sometimes brought up how professionals sometimes see them as problematic as they want to change things "too much" and "too quickly." The resistance from "the cytology side" towards the GCG's cause of removing the Pap smear is a good example here.

References

Akrich, M. (2010), From Communities of Practice to Epistemic Communities: Health Mobilizations on the Internet, *Sociological Research Online*, 15:2, 116–32.

Akrich, M., Leane, M., Roberts, C., and Nunes, J. A. (2014), Practising Childbirth Activism: A Politics of Evidence, *BioSocieties*, 9:2, 129–52.

Armstrong, N., and Eborall, H. (2012), The Sociology of Medical Screening: Past, Present and Future, *Sociology of Health and Illness*, 34:2, 161–76.

Baggott, R., Allsop, J., and Jones, K. (2005), *Speaking for Patients and Carers: Health Consumer Groups and the Policy Process*, Palgrave.

Bloor, K., Hale, V., and Faulkner, A. (2020), Knowledge and Uncertainty in Lyme Disease Detection: An Evidence-Based Activism Research Study in the UK, *Critical Public Health*, doi.org/10.1080/09581596.2019.1704688.

Callon, M. (2009), Elaborating the Notion of Performativity, *Le'Libellio d'AEGIS*, 5:1, 18–29.

Callon, M., and Rabeharisoa, V. (2003), Research "in the Wild" and the Shaping of New Social Identities, *Technology in Society*, 25:2, 193–204.

Cancer Council Australia (2017), *National Cervical Screening Program: Guidelines for the Management of Screen-Detected Abnormalities, Screening in Specific Populations and Investigation of Abnormal Vaginal Bleeding*. Available at: https://wiki.cancer.org.au/australiawiki/images/a/ad/National_Cervical_Screening_Program_guidelines_long-form_PDF.pdf.

Casper, M. J., and Clarke, A. E. (1998), Making the Pap Smear into the "Right Tool" for the Job: Cervical Cancer Screening in the USA, circa 1940–95, *Social Studies of Science*, 28:2, 255–90.

Dahl-Olausson, C. Arvidsson, K. B., Bengtsson, E., Björklin, Å, and Muminovic, E. (2019), Ökningen av cervixcancer—fel att peka ut en hel yrkeskår, *Läkartidningen*, April 1. Available at: https://lakartidningen.se/Opinion/Debatt/2019/01/Okningen-av-cervixcancer–fel-att-peka-ut-en-hel-yrkeskar/.

Dillner, J., Sparén, P., Andrae, B., and Strander, B. (2018), Livmoderhalscancer ökar hos kvinnor med normalt cellprov, *Läkartidningen*, May 6. Available at: http://www.lakartidningen.se/Klinik-och-vetenskap/Rapport/2018/06/Livmoderhalscancer-okar-hos-kvinnor-med-normalt-cellprov/.

Epstein, S. (1996), *Impure Science: AIDS, Activism, and the Politics of Knowledge*, University of California Press.

Epstein, S. (2016), The Politics of Health Mobilization in the United States: The Promise and Pitfalls of "Disease Constituencies," *Social Science and Medicine*, 165, 246–54.

Gill, N., Singleton, V., and Waterton, C. (2017), The Politics of Policy Practices, *Sociological Review*, 65(2_suppl), 3–19.

Hogarth, S., Hopkins, M. M., and Rodriguez, V. (2012), A Molecular Monopoly? HPV Testing, the Pap Smear and the Molecularisation of Cervical Cancer Screening in the USA, *Sociology of Health and Illness*, 34:2, 234–50.

Hogarth, S., Hopkins, M., and Rotolo, D. (2015), Technological Accretion in Diagnostics: HPV Testing and Cytology in Cervical Cancer Screening, in D. Consoli, A. Mina, R. R. Nelson, and R. Ramlogan (eds) *Medical Innovation: Science, Technology and Practice* (88–116), Routledge.

Klawiter, M. (2008), *The Biopolitics of Breast Cancer: Changing Cultures of Disease and Activism*, University of Minnesota Press.

Latour, B. (2004), Why Has Critique Run Out of Steam? From Matters of Fact to Matters of Concern, *Critical Inquiry*, 30:2, 225–48.

Law, J. (2013), Collateral Realities, in P. Baert and F. D. Rubio (eds) *The Politics of Knowledge*, Routledge.

Law, J., and Singleton, V. (2014), ANT, Multiplicity and Policy, *Critical Policy Studies*, 8:4, 379–96.

Lindén, L. (2013), "What Do Eva and Anna Have to Do with Cervical Cancer?" Constructing Adolescent Girl Subjectivities in Swedish Gardasil Advertisements, *Girlhood Studies*, 6:2, 83–100.

Lindén, L. (2017), You Will Protect Your Daughter, Right? In E. Johnson (ed.) *Gendering Drugs: Feminist Studies of Pharmaceuticals* (107–26), Palgrave Macmillan.

Löfgren, H., de Leeuw, E., and Leahy, M. (2011), *Democratizing Health: Consumer Groups in the Policy Process*, Edward Elgar Publishing.

NCI (National Cancer Institute) (2019), *HPV and Pap Testing*. Available at: https://www.cancer.gov/types/cervical/pap-hpv-testing-fact-sheet.

Omni (2018), Australien nära att utrota livmoderhalscancer, *Omni*. Available at: https://omni.se/australien-nara-att-utrota-livmoderhalscancer/a/0Ey2GM.

Panofsky, A. (2011), Generating Sociability to Drive Science: Patient Advocacy Organizations and Genetics Research, *Social Studies of Science*, 41:1, 31–57.

Patient, Consumer, and Public Health Coalition (2014), *Coalition Letter to FDA Commissioner about Approving Cobas HPV Test Alone (without Pap Smear) and FDA Response*. Available at: www.stopcancerfund.org/policy/testimony-briefings/coalition-letter-hpv-test.

Perrone, M. (2014), DNA Alternative to Pap Smear Sparks Medical Debate, *Medical Xpress*, April 15. Available at: https://medicalxpress.com/news/2014-04-dna-alternative-pap-smear-medical.html.

Rabeharisoa, V., Moreira, T., and Akrich, M. (2014a), Evidence-Based Activism: Patients', Users' and Activists' Groups in Knowledge Society, *BioSocieties*, 9:2, 111–28.

Rabeharisoa, V., Callon, M., Filipe, A. M., Nunes, J. A., Paterson, F., and Vergnaud, F. (2014b), From "Politics of Numbers" to "Politics of Singularisation": Patients' Activism and Engagement in Research on Rare Diseases in France and Portugal, *BioSocieties*, 9:2, 194–217.

RCC (Regionala cancercentrum i samverkan) (2019), *Cervixcancerprevention: Nationellt vårdprogram*. Available at: https://www.cancercentrum.se/samverkan/vara-uppdrag/prevention-och-tidig-upptackt/gynekologisk-cellprovskontroll/vardprogram/.

Ronco, G., Giorgi-Rossi, P., Carozzi, F. et al. (2010), Efficacy of Human Papillomavirus Testing for the Detection of Invasive Cervical Cancers and Cervical Intraepithelial Neoplasia: A Randomised Controlled Trial, *The Lancet Oncology*, 11:3, 249–57.

Singleton, V. (1995), Networking Constructions of Gender and Constructing Gender Networks: Considering Definitions of Women in the British Cervical Screening Programme, in K. Grint, R. Gill, and R. M. Gill (eds) *The Gender-Technology Relation: Contemporary Theory and Research* (146–73), Taylor and Francis.

Singleton, V. (1998), Stabilizing Instabilities: The Role of the Laboratory in the United Kingdom Cervical Screening Programme, in M. Berg and A. Mol (eds) *Differences in Medicine: Unravelling Practices, Techniques, and Bodies* (86–104). Duke University Press.

Swedish Cancer Society (2018), *Kraftig ökning av livmoderhalscancer*. Available at: https://www.cancerfonden.se/cancerfondsrapporten/livmoderhalscancer/kraftig-okning-av-livmoderhalscancer.

Tomes, N., and Hoffman, B. (2011), Introduction: Patients as Policy Actors, in B. Hoffman, N. Tomes, R, Grob, and M. Schlesinger (eds) *Patients as Policy Actors: A Century of Changing Markets and Missions* (1–16), Rutgers University Press.

van de Bovenkamp, H. M., Trappenburg, M. J., and Grit, K. J. (2010), Patient Participation in Collective Healthcare Decision Making: The Dutch Model, *Health Expectations*, 13, 1, 73–85.

Wehling, P. (2012), From Invited to Uninvited Participation (and Back?): Rethinking Civil Society Engagement in Technology Assessment and Development, *Poiesis and Praxis*, 9(1–2), 43–60.

7

Heroes, Villains, and Victims

Tracing Breast Cancer Activist Movements

Mohammed Cheded and Gillian Hopkinson

Introduction

Breast cancer, and those affected by breast cancer, have been defined within a contested and fluid terrain. As King (2004, 475) argues, breast cancer has evolved since the 1970s from "a stigmatized disease and individual tragedy best dealt with privately and in isolation, to a neglected epidemic worthy of public debate and political organizing, to an enriching and affirming experience during which women with breast cancer are rarely 'patients' and mostly 'survivors.'" This chapter is concerned with the role that social movement narratives have played in these significant changes in the way that breast cancer is framed, how those with breast cancer are characterized and the consequences that contest between cancer activist movements has on the organization of breast cancer services. This is achieved by examining and contrasting the narratives of diverse movements. It pays particular attention to the metaphoric underpinnings of those narratives and the consequent characterization of women with breast cancer that each seeks to assert and establish in public discourse. We argue that characterization, as portrayed in social movement narratives, has significant consequences both at the individual level as it relates to women's experiences as well as having critical political implications since the dominant characterization has repercussions for the focus of attention and resources, and the way those resources are organized, with respect to the illness.

The chapter focuses on four social movements that provide narrative framings of the terrain of breast cancer. We organize our investigation of these narratives around disease stages. First, we focus on the stage of pre-illness, where we explore (1) the dominant epidemiological narrative and the previvor, and (2) the environmental narrative and the cancerogenic pollutant. Second, we focus on the stages of peri- and post-illness, where we explore

Mohammed Cheded and Gillian Hopkinson, *Heroes, Villains, and Victims: Tracing Breast Cancer Activist Movements*
In: *Healthcare Activism: Markets, Morals, and the Collective Good.* Edited by: Susi Geiger, Oxford University Press.
© Mohammed Cheded and Gillian Hopkinson 2021. DOI: 10.1093/oso/9780198865223.003.0007

166 HEROES, VILLAINS, AND VICTIMS

(3) the pink ribbon narrative and the survivor, and (4) the feminist narrative and the empowered collective. A deeper understanding of these narratives is generated by using a wide variety of publicly available data around breast cancer social movements. These include newspaper articles, novels, memoirs, visual art, online forums and blogs, companies' websites and social media, and journal articles. The relationship between narratives and the consequences of each and their struggle for dominance is interrogated.

The rest of this chapter is structured as follow: first, we flesh out the key concepts underpinning our approach—narrative, characterization, and the social processes/contests amongst multiple narratives. Second, we briefly discuss the disease under study, which is breast cancer, with an emphasis on its cultural hegemony amongst other cancerous diseases. Following that, we move on to discussing the narratives of social movements surrounding breast cancer mentioned above. Through this we are able to contribute in the following ways: first, we highlight the functions of the plotting of the central characters of a social movement narrative and their emotional appeal, in contributing to mobilizing collective action as well as operating as a disciplining tool for the biological citizen. Second, we shed light on the effects of the simplification versus complexification of the characterization of the villain on mobilizing the audience's emotions. Finally, we discuss the role of the individualization and collectivization dynamics in the various social movement narratives in stabilizing and/or destabilizing certain political realities. By doing so, we hope to contribute to developing a better understanding of "the role of literary devices in sociological analyses of collective action" (Polletta 1998, 419).

1. Narratives and Characterization

Social movement narratives in healthcare are important because they contribute to shaping various aspects of the overall disease regime (such as authoritative discourses, emotional discourses, visual imagery, public policies, institutionalized practices, and so on), and subsequently the illness experiences (Klawiter 2004; Willig 2011). As Fine (2002, 244) argues: "by making concrete the theoretical, stories cement individuals into group life emotionally, intellectually, and behaviorally."

According to Fine (2002), social movements constitute a "bundle of narratives." They provide critical cultural resources for connecting the personal and the collective in the experience of injustice against which the need to organize arises. As such, characterization in narratives represents the embodiment of a collective's cultural codes (Jacobs 2002). Social movement narratives can help bridge the gap between the individual and the collective through the construction and reproduction of shared cultures, values, beliefs, as well as commitments to change (Davis 2002; Olsen 2014).

Narratives are essential to mobilizing collective action and thus have a significant impact on the outcomes of social movement activities. As Jacobs (2002, 206) argues, it is through the organization of characters and events into stories that individuals and collectives are able to "develop an understanding of the past, an expectation about the future, and a general understanding of how they should act." A credible narrative requires a logical sequencing of event and emplotment and provides clear linkages between characters and events (Czarniawska 1997). Narrative logic constitutes "powerful devices through which we understand the world" (Hopkinson 2015, 287). These devices are essential to the credibility of a narrative (Polkinghorne 1988). Additionally, narratives provide us, be it explicitly or implicitly, with hints on matters of causality, blame, and accountability (Gabriel 2000). As Fine (2002, 239) put it: "narrative permits the expression of an implicit ideology that even the parties to the discourse may not fully realise is present."

Rather than being a monolithic depiction of events, narratives are fragile and multiple (Bakhtin 1973; Derrida 1979). Storytelling is an active exercise of emplotment, characterization, and sequencing of events, rather than a passive report of what-had-happened. Stories are in competition with each other for establishing credibility and notoriety (Boje 2001). Each story does not operate in isolation but must share the stage with other stories that present alternative accounts, emplotments, and characterization (Hopkinson 2015).

Thus, there is the potential for multiple, and possibly competing, social movement narratives to be present within the same space. In order to mobilize collective action successfully, social movement narratives need to construct an appealing characterization of collective culture so as to claim individuals' allegiance. In addition, social movement narratives should include clear accounts of injustices against which protest must be organized, agents to blame, and measures to monitor the progress of action (Polletta 1998). Collective mobilization requires the identification of an antagonist(s) or a villain(s) within the plot. The arrangement of the relations and interactions between protagonists and antagonists are crucial to creating an engaging plot, which would help mobilize action. As Jacobs (2002, 218) put it, "the narrative ordering of character relations is a strategic resource for social movement leaders."

168   HEROES, VILLAINS, AND VICTIMS

Social movement narratives contribute to redefining dominant conceptions of disease and mobilizing action (Kolker 2004). This chapter explores the construction of dramaturgic characters in narratives of social movements around breast cancer. We present a brief overview of the disease in Section 2.

2. Breast Cancer: A High-Profile Disease

Social movement narratives around breast cancer have been instrumental in mobilizing funding and ultimately shaping the experience of women living with/or at genetic risk of breast cancer. Breast cancer is a high-profile disease due to both its cultural dominance and financial appeal to pharmaceuticals and biotechnology industries. As Ehrenreich (2001, 45) argues, breast cancer has become "the biggest disease on the cultural map, bigger than AIDS, cystic fibrosis, or spinal injury, bigger even than those more prolific killers of women—heart disease, lung cancer and stroke." Breast cancer has high visibility in the media (Clarke and Everest 2006). It has become a highly political disease attracting a large amount of research funding leading some critics to call it "the pinnacle of charitable causes" (King 2004, 473). It enjoys the lion's share of cancer community funding (Klawiter 2008), as well as the largest share of research funding from the most prominent research organizations on cancer such as the United States National Cancer Institute (King 2006). Although in appearance benign (and even positive one could argue), this cultural hegemony has important implications for the construction of women' bodies who are at risk or diagnosed with breast cancer, as well as the framing of other non-mammary related cancers, such as ovarian cancer.

From a financial perspective, breast cancer is a highly lucrative disease. Industry figures highlight how anti-cancer drugs take a clear lead in terms of products in research and development, with a trend showing a steady increase. According to industry, this tendency is here to stay and "cancer's pre-eminence as a therapeutic target . . . is showing all the signs of becoming as immortal as cancer cells themselves" (Pharmaprojects 2019, 14). A ranking of the diseases with the highest number of active drugs in research pipelines shows that "various cancers now account for 14 of the top 20 diseases, and of these, only prostate cancer at number eight and brain cancer at number nine have smaller pipelines this year [2019] than last year [2018]" (Pharmaprojects 2019, 18). Out of these fourteen types of cancer, breast cancer bolsters the largest pipeline with a 6.5 percent increase in the research pipeline between

2018 and 2019. The research pipeline for breast cancer is higher by nearly 33 percent to the second disease in the list, which is lung cancer.

3. Our Method

This chapter draws on a wide variety of North American and United Kingdom sources around breast cancer social movements. These include newspaper articles, novels, memoirs, visual art, online forums and blogs, companies' websites and social media, and journal articles. It is important to emphasize that the chapter does not intend to be an exhaustive review of all the narratives around breast cancer social movements. With the large and ever expanding number of organizations involved in breast cancer social movements, such an endeavor would have been nearly impossible.

We developed our database by following the traces between texts and visuals across times and spaces, and by using online searches primarily. The process was iterative between investigating key social movements around the disease, other central actors that are either explicitly or implicitly involved in the narratives (such as governmental bodies, cosmetic companies, pharmaceutical and biotech companies, and patient support groups), as well as engaging with the relevant literature. Through this iterative process, we were constantly refining our keyword searches. We carried on following the traces between texts and visuals to media coverage, press comments, industry reports, activist group websites and reports, artistic strands of activism such as visual arts and poetry, relevant lawsuits, and so on. The methods for following the traces between texts and visuals was inspired by Izak (2014) (see also Hopkinson 2015). There was no "natural" boundary to the dataset and our snowballing technique to collect it. Thus, we had to make some decisions on the selections of material and the process of tracing the sources and information to the extent that we felt able to present our narrative of the events and draw out key dynamics of characterization of the different narratives of social movements around breast cancer.

During our data analysis, we divided the dataset into two large clusters, each containing two subclusters. The main clusters are organized around the disease stages, while the subclusters are structured around the movement narratives during each stage. The first cluster focuses on the stage of pre-illness and is subdivided into (1) the dominant epidemiological narrative and the previvor, and (2) the environmental narrative and the cancerogenic pollutant. The second cluster focuses on the stages of peri- and post-illness, and is

170 HEROES, VILLAINS, AND VICTIMS

subdivided into (1) the pink ribbon narrative and the survivor, and (2) the feminist narrative and the empowered collective.

After a first round of exploration of material around breast cancer social movements' narrative, we selected, within each cluster, examples that revolve around the themes of aesthetics and the body, empowerment, funding and access, survivorship, previvorship, responsibility(ies), individualization, collectivization, biomedical orthodoxies, and alternative forms and modes of knowledge. The data analysis primarily draws on insights from discursive psychology (Potter and Wetherell 1987), with particular attention given to the matters of attribution of blame, causality, and responsibility (Edwards and Potter 1993). The analysis of visual material was largely inspired by Van Leeuwen's (1993) multi-modal discourse analysis. The analysis is presented in Section 4.

4. Analysis

4.1 Social Movement Narratives around Pre-Illness

The initial experiences of women living with breast cancer have often been described as "relentlessly individualised" and characterized by "stigma, isolation and invisibility" (Klawiter 2004, 865–6). The experiences of breast cancer as an individual journey filled with stigma are further exacerbated by the dominant epidemiological narrative of cancer as a disease occasioned by the self. Heredity, genetics, age, and lifestyle are frequently positioned at the top of the list of risk factors for cancer in biomedical and popular discourses (see for example Centre for Disease Control 2018). Framing cancer as a disease occasioned by the self has important political effects. One such notable effect is that it sets other framings to the background, such as the political framing which focuses for instance on the relationship between inequalities and the incidence of cancer, or the environmental framing which emphasizes the role of environmental contaminants (Brown et al. 2001; Kolker 2004). Furthermore, disease framing has important implications for determining the sites of responsibility and blame, which in turn favors the legitimization of particular tools of control that are deemed appropriate to target the source of blame—i.e. the self in this case. We focus next on social movements around the BRCA gene and breast cancer as a genetic disease to illustrate the characterization work in the dominant epidemiological narratives.

4.1.1 The Dominant Epidemiological Narrative and the Previvor

Within the dominant epidemiological narrative, the etiology of the disease is often linked to the individual. Whether it is family, history, genetics, age, lifestyle, breast density, or reproductive history, the construction of breast cancer as "a disease 'occasioned' by the self" incriminates the patient in the a etiology of the disease, as Stacey (1997, 175) put it. The genetics narrative reinforces the individualistic construction of both the disease and the experiences of women who are labelled "at genetic risk" for breast cancer. Inheriting a mutation in BRCA1 and BRCA2 is considered to be linked to an increased risk of female breast and ovarian cancers. The BRCA1 and BRCA2 mutations account for about 20 percent of hereditary breast cancer, around 5 to 10 percent of all breast cancers, and approximately 15 percent of all ovarian cancers (Pal et al. 2005; National Cancer Institute 2015). Despite these fairly low figures, breast cancer is probably the most geneticized type of cancer. Furthermore, the labeling of the gene is related to breast cancer only, as BRCA is an acronym for BReast CAncer, and the genes are known as BReast CAncer 1 (BRCA1) and BReast CAncer 2 (BRCA2). This is what led the gene to be commonly known as the breast cancer gene, despite being associated with other types of cancer. The genetic determinism surrounding breast cancer has had dramatic effects with regards to the media coverage of the BRCA gene as well as the social movement narratives surrounding it—with the most notable being the objectification and emphasis of breast cancer as a disease occasioned by the self.

There is a particularly interesting characterization of patients that takes center stage within the geneticized breast cancer movement narratives: the *previvor*. The term previvor was coined on the forum of the online biosocial community FORCE to describe the experiences of women living with a BRCA mutation. We will introduce FORCE in further detail when discussing the role of online biosocial communities as supporting devices for plotting the social movement narrative of the previvor, but let's focus on the characterization of the previvor for now. The FORCE website defines the identifier "previvor" as follows:

"Cancer previvors" are individuals who are sur*vivors* of a *pre*disposition to *cancer* but who haven't had the disease. This group includes people who carry a hereditary mutation, a family history of cancer, or some other predisposing factor. The cancer previvor term evolved from a challenge on the FORCE main message board by . . . a website regular, who posted, "I need a label!" As a result, the term *cancer previvor* was chosen to identify those

172 HEROES, VILLAINS, AND VICTIMS

living with risk. The term specifically applies to the portion of our community which has its own unique needs and concerns separate from the general population, but different from those already diagnosed with cancer.

The medical community uses the term "unaffected carrier" to describe those who have not had cancer but have a BRCA or other cancer-predisposing mutation. The term applies from a medical perspective, but doesn't capture the experience of those who face an increased risk for cancer and the need to make medical management decisions. Although cancer previvors face some of the same fears as cancer survivors, undergoing similar tests and confronting similar medical management issues, they face a unique set of emotional, medical, and privacy concerns.

(FORCE, © FORCE-Facing Our Risk of Cancer Empowered, Inc.,
Tampa, Florida. All rights reserved)

While the term refers to a predisposition to cancer in a broad sense, it is often used to discuss "cancer-predisposing mutations" and the BRCA gene predominantly. The previvor has a predisposition to breast cancer and knows of her propensity. She is in a liminal category of wellness, as she is "neither actually ill (yet) nor fully well" (Lupton 2012, 17). She is said to be empowered to navigate her diagnosis by engaging with biomedical knowledge around genomics. Through this engagement, she is empowered to receive genetic screening, educate herself, and monitor her breasts for malignancies in order to make informed choices that help control her risk to develop cancer. Thus, the previvor represents an empowered risky subject. She is a science-literate patient/consumer who is willing to make use of the resources available to make an "informed choice." The internet has been a driver for the shaping of the "informed/empowered" patient. The plethora of web-based health-related information is said to enable the education of patients, while the online forums provide space for support, information, and story sharing. This process of education, which is primarily concerned with the compliance with biomedical orthodoxy, allows for this form of empowerment of consumers of preventive healthcare services to be possible.

What is striking here is the alignment of empowerment goals with biomedical orthodoxy and individualization trends in healthcare (Geiger and Gross 2017; Geiger 2020), as well as notions of responsibilization and self-care (Beckmann 2013). Later in this analysis, we will explore the original forms of patient empowerment in breast cancer movement narratives, when discussing feminist social movement narratives. Next, we further illustrate the characterization work of the previvor in our analysis of the supporting plotting devices for the dominant epidemiological narrative.

4.1.1.1 Supporting Devices for Plotting the Social Movement Narrative of the Previvor

Mass media: Mass media has constituted an essential device for plotting the social movement narrative of the *previvor*. There have been several popular figures who have gone public, in the past decade, about their mastectomies (whether curative or preventive). Just to name a few: Christina Applegate, Olivia Newton-John, Lynn Redgrave, Katy Bates, and Sharon Osbourne all announced their medical choices to the public. Sharon Osbourne, for instance, revealed to *Hello!* magazine that she undertook a preventive double mastectomy after discovering that she had "the breast-cancer gene" (Hellomagazine.com 2012). In addition, there was another key piece that sparked a tremendous interest in the BRCA gene. The article was written by the American actress, film director, screenwriter, and author Angelina Jolie, and published in the *New York Times* on May 14, 2013. In her piece entitled "My Medical Choice," Angeline Jolie revealed to the public her decision to undertake a double mastectomy following her diagnosis as a faulty gene carrier. The article sparked enormous interest, both in terms of media coverage and reaction, as well as public interest. The public interest went beyond the revelation of Angelina Jolie onto knowing more about the faulty gene.

The most notable headline that followed Angelina Jolie's article was the "The Angelina Effect," which was the cover of the *Time* on May 27, 2013. The term was initially used to describe the "cultural and medical earthquake" caused by the star's revelation. A study appearing in the journal *Breast Cancer Research* in 2014 revealed that "the Angelina effect" more than doubled the frequency of testing for the BRCA gene in the United Kingdom following the publication of the letter (Evans et al. 2014). Similar studies were conducted in other Western countries such as Australia and Canada, revealing a similar tendency to increased screening (CBC News 2013; Hagan 2013). Another study published in the *British Medical Journal* in 2016 showed that "the Angelina effect" has indeed caused a significant increase in testing, but not in mastectomy rates. The authors argue that the information might not have reached the population that is "really" at risk and just participated in increasing the paranoia surrounding genetic diseases (Desai and Jena 2016). The piece represents an individualized form of activism around the BRCA gene and the risky subject. However, the notoriety and credibility of the narrator definitely increased the impact of the story in this case. As Benford and Snow

(2000, 621) put it: "the greater the status and/or perceived expertise of the frame articulator and/or the organization they represent from the vantage point of potential adherents and constituents, the more plausible and resonant the framings or claims."

Throughout the piece, the dichotomy hope/fear plays an important role in the characterization work of the previvor. The narrative of fear is set from the outset, with metaphors of war such as "MY MOTHER fought cancer for almost a decade and died at 56" (capitalization in original). It is also discernible through metaphors of the invisible, yet omnipresent danger in "living *under the shadow* of cancer" (emphasis added). Another device at the service of this narrative is the use of factual descriptions of risk, with the example of "My doctors estimated that I had an 87 percent risk of breast cancer and a 50 percent risk of ovarian cancer." The narrative emphasizes the "reality" of the risk associated with carrying a BRCA gene mutation and the amplitude of the danger accompanying it. This can be seen for example in "I have always told them [her children] not to worry, but the truth is I carry a 'faulty' gene, BRCA1, which sharply increases my risk of developing breast cancer and ovarian cancer." The previvor is aware of her risk. She is also science-literate and able to make sense of the statistics available to her. In addition, the previvor is fearful of what might happen. The source of fear is a quantified, credible statistic made available to her through genetic screening. The adjective "risky" of the "empowered risky subject" materializes through the quantification and objectification of risk. Thus, the previvor is fearful of what is yet to come. The prophecy of her fate is written in her character name, and evidenced by "objective" science.

Power and empowerment are also key themes in the letter. These themes are used to set the scene in line with the narratives of fear, in for example "Cancer is still a word that strikes fear into people's hearts, producing a deep sense of *powerlessness*" (emphasis added). They are also positioned as a response to the narratives of danger and fear. The argument of "empowerment"-as-a-solution is visible from the title of the article itself, "My Medical Choice," which signals ownership of medical destiny and the responsibility to preserve the body. The previvor is not only aware of her risk, but also willing and able to make an informed choice based on the options available to her. This can be seen, for instance, in Angelina's statement "once I knew that this was my reality, I decided to be proactive and to minimise the risk as much as I could." The previvor is responsibilized for taking back control over her risk.

The empowerment is visible in the narrative of ownership of the medical destiny and risk reduction. It also transpires through a restitution narrative that is very similar to those present in the survivorship discourse. In narrating her post-reconstructive surgery, Angelina states "they [her children] can see my small scars and that's it. Everything else is *just* Mommy, the same as she always was' (emphasis added). Here, she asserts control over her risk, and thereby her "identity" and "self" through the control of body image by means of reconstitutive surgery. The faulty genes and defective organs are constructed as "other" to the self. What remains of this "other" after the preventive surgery is the "small scars" only. The scars are reminiscent of the defective organ. However, the subject position "Mommy" is stabilized through the qualification of the scars as "small," therefore limiting their effects. This positions stereotypical and gendered responsibilities as central to the decision to preserve the body. The previvor can and should seek to reconstruct her heterofeminine body. Otherwise, she risks losing her womanhood because of the removal of her breasts.

Online biosocial communities: Online spaces constitute another important device for plotting the social movement narrative of the previvor. These spaces include, but are not limited to, forums, blogs, patient support groups, and so on. Their digital nature helps bring together communities that can be geographically dispersed, such as the communities of carriers of BRCA gene mutations. These online spaces often reproduce elements from the discourse of survivorship, which is akin to peri- and post-illness narratives. This is visible through the usage of "branded" breast cancer colors, for example, vivid pink.

While a lot of these spaces focus on patients' support and narratives, some bring together a variety of actors such as healthcare practitioners, genetics and cancer researchers, alongside patient advocacy groups. FORCE constitutes an example of an organization which enrolls several actors around a genetic mutation. Another notable aspect of FORCE is the bridging between the online and offline, as it holds its own annual conference that gathers healthcare practitioners, genetics and cancer researchers, patient advocacy groups and patients, as well as frequently advertising clinical trials for members to enroll in. Rabinow (1992) anticipated the emergence of such collectives, describing them as "biosocial communities." He envisaged that such groups would form around "new truths" produced by the Human Genome Project and outlined the requirements for such movements to materialize. These requirements included the organization of efforts around specific DNA mutations and the mobilization of genetic experts, medical specialists, laboratories, diagnostic technologies, narratives, and support groups. Collectively these features allow previvors to "understand" and

176 HEROES, VILLAINS, AND VICTIMS

deal with an almost determined fate of disease development caused by that mutation (Pender 2012).

While her responsibility is individual, the previvor organizes collectively with other women who share her genetic identity. They gather to support but also monitor each other. Peer monitoring has critical effects on the characterization work. It implicitly sets the stage for protagonists and antagonists within the narrative. While the protagonist/hero is personified in the previvor who is an empowered risky subject, the antagonist/villain manifests in the *irresponsible risky subject*. The irresponsible risky subject does not comply with biomedical rationalities around the dominant epidemiological model. She does not take care of herself as per the guidelines, lacks awareness about her genetic risk and its implications, and exposes herself to known risk factors. In order to legitimize their membership to the collective of previvors, individuals have to avoid falling into the category of the irresponsible risky subject. This was visible in the politics of advice giving and receiving in online forums, where women were carefully crafting a narrative of their stories prior to asking for advice. In the extract below from a forum discussion board dedicated to BRCA-positive women, a participant attempts to legitimize her reluctance to undertake the preventive surgery by establishing a causal link between menopause-inducing surgery and her subsequent ability to provide care for her small children. Such crafting of the narrative was necessary for the forum participant to legitimize questioning biomedical rationalities without being labeled irresponsible.

> I will most definitely ask about breast cancer risk. I have no problem having a mastectomy, to be honest if that's what the doctor recommends. The hysterectomy scares me due to the potential body changes, hormone problems, mood issues, etc. This is mainly because I have small children. If I didn't have kids to take care of, I wouldn't care about that so much either. (Forum participant)

This binary of responsibility has important implications for collective dynamics. The arrangement of characters of a narrative in a binary relationship (antagonist and protagonist), has significant effects on the evaluative and dramatic intensity of the narrative (Jacobs 2002). Such plotting contributes to praising the previvor for her courage and determination to take control over her risk. By the same token, it frames the irresponsible risky subject as negligent and casts her back into the shadow. The spotlight is put on the previvor, which bears similarities to the narrative of survivorship, explored below.

4.1.2 The Environmental Movement Narrative and the Cancerogenic Pollutant

The environmental movement has challenged biomedical and popular explanations of causality of breast cancer—particularly with regards to an emphasis on personal lifestyle and genetics. At the center of the environmental narrative is the situated understanding of the epidemiology of breast cancer, and a commitment to shed light on the corporate and governmental responsibility in the etiology of the disease. As Rothman (1998, 169) put it: "the social epidemiology of cancer, the role of industrial capitalism, gets glossed over as the cancer moves deeper and deeper inside the individual." The environmental movement attempts to disrupt this ideology by re-emphasizing the role of industrial capitalism.

In order to challenge the dominant epidemiological narrative and destabilize the center of blame, the environmental movement has tackled the scientific approach to researching breast cancer. It has been committed to decentering the biomedical model that focused on individualistic methods for research, treating, and preventing cancer, by drawing attention to the health effects of environmental pollutants. The environmental movement aims to shape both research and policy to a focus on environmental causes of breast cancer, as well as increase public awareness towards these issues. Since its inception in the early 1990s (Zavestoski et al. 2004; Klawiter 2008), the environmental movement has been committed to scrutinizing the effects of cancerogenic pollutants as well as the political, economic, and social structures that allowed such exposures to occur. To this end, the movement has pushed the role of transdisciplinary research models in order to include a broader spectrum of disciplines and actors in the understanding of the epidemiology of breast cancer (Osuch et al. 2012).

Environmental narratives displace the blame and responsibility from its individualized conceptualization within the dominant epidemiological narrative, onto corporations and government structures responsible for the exposure of women to cancerogenic pollutants. By doing so, they debunk the myth of the previvor/empowered risky subject as the solution to preventing breast cancer and expose the complexities of breast cancer causality to the public. Rather than relying on a simplified narrative, such as the case with the dominant epidemiological narrative (Sulik 2014), environmental narratives encourage expert and laypeople alike to acknowledge and explore the

178   HEROES, VILLAINS, AND VICTIMS

intricacies inherent to breast cancer causality and investigate the accountability of corporations and government structures for the exposure of women to cancer-causing agents. Thus, these institutions take the lead villain role within this narrative.

The villain character is overall depicted as dark, mischievous, but also full of mystery. On the one hand, the overall lack of knowledge around environmental contaminants and the causal mechanisms involved in the process participates in reinforcing both dimensions of harm and mystery. The source of harm is lurking in the background. On the other hand, the language used to describe the process of exposure participates in the de/mystification of the character of the villain. The usage of both nominalization and passivation is widespread in the mainstream narratives around the exposure to environmental pollutants. Biomedical narratives focus on discussing the effects of "environmental/chemical exposure," "individual's exposure," "lifetime exposure," and so on. On the other hand, environmental activist narratives specify the focus of the effects of such exposition on their impact on women's livelihoods, as well as vulnerable communities. The two extracts below from Breast Cancer Action's factsheet on breast cancer and the environment highlight such focus.

> We cannot put the burden on consumers to buy "safer" products. Below are examples of some of the ways *we are routinely exposed.* (Emphasis added)
>
> Disadvantaged populations, especially communities of color, are more likely to be employed in occupations with higher levels of toxic chemical exposure such as manufacturing, agriculture, and certain service sector occupations. They are also more likely to live in more highly contaminated communities. Studies have shown that these unequal exposures result in racial and ethnic differences in chemical body burdens of certain chemicals such as flame retardants, BPA and phthalates.

The usage of nominalization and passivization performs the function of deleting agency and reifying processes (Fowler et al. 1979; Billig 2008). In this case, the process of hiding agency is either intentional (protecting the agent) or constrained by legal boundaries (insufficient evidence to incriminate the agent).

When the evidence against the institutions responsible for the exposure to cancerogenic pollutants is possible, the language adapts, and the layer of mystery of the character unveils to reveal dark and mischievous attributes. For instance in 2018, the organization Earthjustice represented a coalition of health, consumer, and environmental activist organizations in a lawsuit aimed at pressuring the United States Food and Drug Administration (FDA) to prohibit cancerogenic artificial chemicals widely used for food flavoring. The petitioners represented were Breast Cancer Prevention Partners, Center for Environmental Health, Center for Food Safety, Center for Science in the Public Interest, Environmental Defense Fund, Environmental Working Group, Natural Resources Defense Council, and WE ACT for Environmental Justice. The chemicals at issue in the lawsuit are benzophenone, ethyl acrylate, eugenyl methyl ether, myrcene, pulegone, pyridine, and styrene. They are recognized to be widely used to flavor baked goods, ice cream, candy, and so on. The legal document clearly frames the responsibility and failure of the FDA to act on these widely used cancerogenic chemicals. As the senior strategic advisor of Earthjustice states: "consumers cannot identify every ingredient in processed food and they shouldn't have to; we need FDA to do its job and protect our health and welfare."

4.1.2.1 Supporting Devices for Plotting the Social Movement Narrative of the Cancerogenic Pollutant
Seeing that environmental causality is the least mentioned topic in media coverage of breast cancer (Zavestoski et al. 2004), activist campaigns constitute the main terrain for the plotting of the environmental narrative. An example of such campaigns is "Think Before You Pink" launched by Breast Cancer Action (a key organization of feminist cancer activism) launched in 2002. Think Before You Pink campaigns to expose corporations' *pink-washing* practices and encourages consumers to be critical and reflexive about their consumption of pink ribbon products. The campaign targeted the practices within the mainstream breast cancer movement around the pink ribbon, which we explore in depth later in the chapter. It highlighted how some cosmetics product that are part of the pink ribbon campaigns contain known cancerogenic chemicals that can increase the risk of breast cancer.

In 2013 the Breast Cancer Fund and the *Campaign for Safe Cosmetics* reviewed products from the cosmetic giant Revlon. They discovered the presence of toxic and cancerogenic components hormone-disturbing chemicals such as titanium dioxide (a respiratory carcinogen), carbon black, and polyacrylamide (which may contain traces of mammary carcinogen). The products were part of the "Revlon Cares" program, with the slogan "Your lips can save lives." This is not an isolated incident, as the cosmetics industry has had close ties with the breast cancer mainstream movement, flooding the market with pink ribbon-derived products such as lipstick, nail polish,

180 HEROES, VILLAINS, AND VICTIMS

perfume, and so on. Environmental campaigns, such as Think Before You Pink contribute to the processes of debunking the altruistic façade of certain corporations, as well as centering the corporations and government structures, responsible for the exposure of women to cancerogenic pollutants, as the lead villain character of this narrative.

The overall language of causation is important to the characterization work as well. While dominant epidemiological narratives discuss how cancer cells are made instead of born within (Steingraber 1997), environmental narratives shift the locus of blame to cancer-causing chemicals, as well as the political, economic, and social structures that allowed exposures to the causal agent to occur. This has an effect not only on the characterization of the villain but also on the overall plotting. As such, the hope for deliverance of the disease is no longer narrated in terms of controlling individual risk factors but through the lens of hope for alternative ways of understanding and doing breast cancer care. As Potts (2004, 133) argues, there is "a 'transformational vision' of the physical, political, social and economic environments that currently contribute to breast cancer."

By doing so, environmental narratives propose an ideological repositioning of the very conceptualization of "risk" when discussing breast cancer. Primary cancer prevention is achieved through the identification and elimination of the "causes" or "risk factors" leading to the development of cancer (Fosket 2010). Hence it is crucial to act on the understanding of the processes of calculation and qualification of risk factors for breast cancer, and shift them from a sole focus on the individual to include the collective risk. Next, we move onto analyzing social movement narratives around peri- and post-illness.

4.2 Social Movement Narratives around Peri- and Post-Illness

There have historically been two major distinct approaches to breast cancer activism around the stages of peri- and post-illness. On the one hand, there is activism focused essentially on fundraising. This strand has worked towards the destigmatization of the disease, as well as fundraising for research, screening, and education. It has also contributed strongly to shaping the treatments, the screening methods, and the number of spaces for support available for patients. The mobilization around the pink ribbon is a great example of such activism. However, this type of activism does not necessarily challenge the conventional approaches of its areas of action (research, screening, and education), as has been pointed out by feminist critiques (King 2004; Klawiter

2008). On the other hand, feminist activism has been geared towards political action. The primary purpose of these activists is to destabilize the dominant methods of understanding and acting on breast cancer. Some of the major topics that it addresses are the blurring of the lines between prevention and early detection, as well as issues of access to the marginalized such as poor people, ethnic minorities, disabled, and LGBT women.

4.2.1 The Pink Ribbon Narrative and the Survivor

Much of the mainstream narrative around peri-illness sets the scene for the central character of post-illness, that is the "survivor." The mainstream narrative swings between two domains primarily: the body as a battlefield and the hope for a cure. While the former is concerned with the individualized experience, the latter focuses on biomedical victories. Another notable difference is the emotional charge, with the former revolving around fear and the latter around hope. These domains are connected through the umbrella theme of "fight against breast cancer."

Fighting, war, and battlefield constitute essential metaphorical formulations in breast cancer narratives that are central to the plotting and characterization work of the narrative. "War" metaphors are pervasive within cancer narratives (Sontag 1978). The human body becomes the battlefield, and the language of treatment is centered on fighting against a deadly, insidious enemy. The biomedical literature talks about "bombarding" areas of the body with radiation, or treatment aiming at "killing" cancer cells. Metaphors in breast cancer possess an overtly politicized character. The metaphors of war are not purely linguistic embellishments—they actually shape practices. As Annas (1997, 68) states: "military thinking concentrates on the physical, sees control as central, and encourages the expenditure of massive resources to achieve dominance."

However, the "star" of mainstream narratives is incontestably the *survivor*. The domain of battlefield and fight against breast cancer sets the stage for the primary functions of mainstream narrative: the "hope" for a cure which requires funding, and the celebration of biomedical successes and survivors. The survivor represents this figure of hope from within the collective, who "made it" to the other side. The narrative is straightforward: "in order to have more survivors, we need a cure. And in order to find a cure, we need funding!"

4.2.1.1 Supporting Devices for Plotting the Social Movement Narrative of the Survivor

Marketing campaigns, media coverage, social media: The hope for a cure is the primary driver for research, and the necessity to generate funding in order

182 HEROES, VILLAINS, AND VICTIMS

to achieve this aim. Approaches to generate funding have been very diverse. Some of the primary activities of this movement are focused on generating funding to support research, which will hopefully lead to funding a cure for breast cancer. These activities range from all the pink ribbon-branded products (such as *Estée Lauder's Breast Cancer Awareness range),* different fundraising races and marathons (such as the Susan G. Komen Foundation's Race for the Cure), or the MacMillan free kits for fundraising events in the United Kingdom. The symbolism of the mainstream breast cancer activist movement through a vivid pink-colored ribbon was a surprising choice at first. Indeed, pink is a color constructed in our contemporary culture as girly, pretty, and healthy, which makes it an odd choice for a disease such as breast cancer that is characterized by a loss of womanhood (King 2006). Nevertheless, the cultural construction of the color pink functions as a device for the materialization of the overly positive tone of the survivorship discourse. The survivor is optimistic, upbeat, and positive. She is also feminine, girly, and bubbly.

The latest campaign from *Estée* Lauder carries the legacy of this colorful and optimistic tone. The slogan of the fall 2018–19 campaign was "time to end breast cancer," with a trending hashtag on Instagram and Twitter #TimeToEndBreastCancer. We analyzed the "top" posts attached to the hashtag on Instagram (in terms of likes) out of a total of 14,038 posts at the time of writing this chapter (September 2019). Our examination highlighted that alongside the "girly, pretty, and healthy," the glamorous takes center stage. The theme of glamor has been present within breast cancer social movements for over a couple of decades now. For example, in 1996 the *New York Times* qualified breast cancer movements as the "Year's Hot Charity" (Belkin 1996). The same year, the fashion model Linda Evangelista was the face of an important breast cancer awareness campaign. The visual was a head and shoulders shot of Evangelista, coiffed with her iconic haircut at the time, and with her left arm across her chest, covering her breast in a much stylized fashion pose. The narrative of the *New York Times* piece was centered on the willingness of corporations and politicians to support the cause, thanks to the work of activists and survivors on the cultural appeal of breast cancer. Thus, the survivor is glamourous as well. She is appealing culturally and visually, and thus constitutes a figure to be aspired to.

Another notorious example of the mainstream breast cancer social movements is the Breast Cancer Research Stamp that was unveiled by Hillary Clinton in 1998. The slogan of the stamp's campaign was "Fund the fight, find a cure." There are several interesting linguistic devices within this slogan. First of all, the fight is formulated as defined, and the cure as unknown. This is visible through the use of the determiners "the" and "a," respectively. Furthermore, the ordering of the sentence alludes to a causal mechanism between the acts of funding the "fight" and finding a cure; *finding a cure* is constructed as a direct consequence of *funding the fight*. It also constructs the act of *finding a cure* as a collective act.[1] This specific formulation has a function of framing the "right" ways of fighting breast cancer as established and somewhat indisputable, and the cure as a subsequent collective effort that is contingent on the funding of the fight. Such practices construct survivorship and cure as individual acts of philanthropy performed within the arena of consumer culture (King 2004). The survivor is compassionate and demonstrates this virtue through consumption practices.

Feminist critiques have pointed out the profound political effects of the practices surrounding the survivorship movement, and suggest viewing them as an exercise of the fulfillment of obligations as part of the individual's *biological citizenship* (Petryna 2004; Rose and Novas 2005; Kerr et al. 2009). Biological citizenship refers to a new kind of citizenship, which emerged with the rapid progress of biomedical research, genomics, and biotechnology. This citizenship is shaped by new subjectivities, politics, and ethics (Rose and Novas 2005). The new forms of biosocial groups organize around shared biomarkers (the online biosocial communities discussed in this chapter constitute an example of such groups). They stake claims to specific rights while sharing a set of duties and responsibilities as part of their biosocial membership (Kerr et al. 2009). The model figure of the biological citizen is framed as a compassionate consumer, but also a consumer of compassion, who is actively involved in philanthropic programs in an effort to strive to become the *ideal* biological citizen. Survivors are depicted as "courageous, self-responsible, high-order citizens" (King 2004, 489). However, this biological citizen does not challenge established methods of organizing against breast cancer. Her duties are delineated into securing funding, volunteering in events, and participating in clinical trials when applicable. Bell (2014, 62) views biological citizenship within the breast cancer movement as "the subsequent willingness of white, middle-class women with a history of breast cancer to participate in research as part of their perceived duties as 'good' biological citizens."

4.2.2 The Feminist Narrative and the Empowered Collective

Parallel to the mainstream breast cancer movement, feminist cancer activism was committed to providing a space for the unheard voices. Taking inspiration from the LGBT movement around AIDS, this movement has been challenging the upbeat discourse of survivorship. The movement has also questioned the centricity of the character "survivor." Indeed, the core principles of the model of AIDS activism was the organization of the fight against the demonization of people affected by AIDS. Yet, the movement was equally dismissive of the trivialization of the condition through overly positive messages. Similarly, feminist cancer activism is critical of the normalization of women bodies who are affected by breast cancer. Whilst the mainstream breast cancer movement promoted unscarred, heterofeminine—albeit cancerized—bodies, feminist activists championed making spaces available for the expression of "alternative images, alternative discourses, and alternative ways of embodying breast cancer" (Klawiter 2008, 169). Indeed, survivorship stories put forward what Frank (1995) calls a "restitution narrative," where the character who re-emerges at the end of the cancer journey is reconstructed in a way to embody heterofeminine notions of womanhood still. Such a scenario is possible thanks to the heroic acts of fighting by the survivor, as well as the technologies of reconstruction. Through technologies of the body such as breast reconstruction, prostheses, wigs, and a careful choice of clothing, the transformation of breast cancer survivors' bodies so that they can mirror the image of healthy ones is not only made possible but encouraged within the survivorship discourse. Feminist activism highlights how the dominant discourse of survivorship actually distorts the ugly realities of the experiences of women living with breast cancer. Instead of the "normalized" body, the feminist movements gave a space for the scarred, the one-breasted, and unbreasted bodies, as well as other non-conformist and marginalized identities. It "celebrated the ongoing struggles of women 'living with cancer'" (Klawiter 2008, 169), rather than the overly positive image of cancer survivors. Thus, the central character of this narrative is the collective affected by the disease. It is a collective that is characterized by its diversity, and hosts many of those deemed "misfits" by society.

The feminist movement dedicated its efforts also to mobilizing support, care, and compassion for women living with cancer, especially the marginalized such as disabled, LGBT, ethnic minorities, and poor women. Mostly, feminist breast cancer activism was committed to a culture of patient empowerment. Empowerment is understood, within this context, as giving voice to expressions of sorrow, anger, grief, and other unpleasant emotions to those who were alienated by the survivorship discourse.

It is crucial at this stage to clearly delineate the meanings and usage of "empowerment" in this context, as it has important implications for the characterization of the "empowered collective," which is very distinct from the "empowered risky subject" (previvor). Empowerment is a polysemic term and has had some contradictory applications, including in the case of breast cancer activism. The initial culture of patient empowerment in feminist activist movements in healthcare did draw on the activist movement within HIV/AIDS in the gay community (Klawiter 2008), and its meaning and applications were linked to the origins of the term. "Empowerment" can be traced to the 1976 publication of "Black Empowerment: Social Work in Oppressed Communities" by Barbara Solomon, where the term started to be formally used in research and social services (Calvès 2009). Its early usage signaled a commitment to giving a voice to the oppressed, enabling them to fight against the dominating voices to which they were subjected. The empowerment was then said to be realized through a movement from a "dominated consciousness" to a "critical consciousness" (Freire 1974). The primary tools described in these early versions were education, particularly in relation to issues of domination, through the deconstruction of dominant constructs such as race and gender. The influences were very diverse, and included Freudian psychology, feminism, the Black Power movement, and Gandhism (Sharma 2008). It was in the mid-1980s that the term empowerment started to gain increasing popularity, promoted by the feminist movement. This influence spread to the field of international development, which constituted a platform for the term to infiltrate policy and program documents pervasively (Calvès 2009). Despite the diverse influences, the focus of empowerment at the time was still addressing issues of inequality and domination; hence its suitable application in the early feminist activist movements for breast cancer. The empowered collective is critical of issues of access associated with structural inequalities. They are also motivated by the anger resulting from the inequality and injustice that some of their members might face. Furthermore, they are skeptical of the mainstream movements and their potential complicity with structures of domination.

4.2.2.1 Supporting Devices for Plotting the Social Movement Narrative of the Empowered Collective

Visual art, memoirs, and politics: Visual art, memoirs, and mass media were strong mediums for the dissemination of feminist movement narratives. One of the most notable examples is the portrait of the breast cancer activist and artist Matuschka, which made quite an impact when it featured in the *New York Times Magazine* in 1993. The image was a self-portrait and clearly displayed a mastectomy scar in the original location of her right breast. The top-right part of the dress was cut in such a way as to make a statement with this visual. The headline reads: "You Can't Look Away Anymore: The

186 HEROES, VILLAINS, AND VICTIMS

Anguished Politics of Breast Cancer" (Ferraro 1993). The narrative of the article was very much influenced by feminist activism, addressing issues of prevention, public awareness, as well as the linkages between environmental contaminants and disease incidence rates. The tone of the image and article contrasts dramatically with the title discussed earlier proclaiming breast cancer as the "year's hot charity," which appeared only three years later in the *New York Times Magazine* (Belkin 1996). The previous image of the scarred body, which was described by some readers as "shock therapy" (Anonymous 1993), left the space to a photograph of Linda Evangelista analyzed in the previous section.

The self-portrait of Matuschka entitled "Beauty out of Damage" was part of a movement of visual art which contributed to the visibility of the struggles of women living with breast cancer from the 1970s to the 1990s. One of the most notable examples of that era is a portrait of the American poet Deena Metzger exhibiting a tattooed mastectomy scar. The poster featured a photograph taken by Hella Hammid and a poem written by Deena Metzger. We present a short extract from the poem, which features in Metzger's book *Tree: Essays and Pieces* (1997):

> I am no longer afraid of mirrors where I see the sign of the amazon,
> the one who shoots arrows.
> There was a fine red line across my chest where a knife entered, but
> now a branch winds about the scar and travels from arm to heart.

The theme of war and battle are central to Metzger's poem (and photograph). However, their usage is different from mainstream breast cancer movements. In this instance, the metaphors of war function as devices for the celebration of the scarred and unbreasted female body. This inclusion of alternative cancerous bodies helps us relate to the struggle of women living with cancer, which contrasts with the overly optimistic mainstream narrative that focused on survivorship and the reconstruction of the heteronormative. Other examples of visual art as a medium for representing breast cancer include "Marked Up for Amputation" by British educational photographer Jo Spence (1995), and the collection of painting *Breast Cancer Journal* by Holli Sigler (1999) illustrating her experience of living with breast cancer. The empowered collective does not shy away from the ugly truths of living with breast cancer. Instead, they mobilize the emotions of anger that can stem from looking at these realities, and utilize them as fuel to organize action.

Alongside visual art, breast cancer memoirs have been a popular medium for representing the struggles of living with breast cancer. Amongst the most notable contributions are Rose Kushner's *Breast Cancer: A Personal History and an Investigative Report* (1975), Susan Sontag's *Illness as Metaphor* (1978), and André Lorde's *The Cancer Journals* (1980). They have addressed topics such as the environmental causes of breast cancer, the stigmatization of cancer patients, and the struggle of minorities living with cancer such as those of black women and LGBT women. Breast cancer feminist narratives have also challenged hegemonic models of communication about cancer such as the military metaphors in cancer care, as well as the obsession with the restitution of the heteronormative body through reconstructive surgery (Frank 1995). Moreover, these narratives confronted the corporate complicity with mainstream cancer activism, and more recently challenged genetic testing on the grounds of ethics, access, and efficacy (DeShazer and Helle 2014). The empowered collective embraces alternative forms of representation. They mobilize their anger for a fight for broader access. The fight is collective, which contrasts with the survivor's fight against a disease occasioned by the self. It is a fight against the political and social structures that generate and reproduce inequalities of access to healthcare.

5. Discussion

To start our discussion, we summarize in Table 7.1 the list of dramatis personae as featured in the social movement narratives analyzed in this

Table 7.1 Summary of the dramatis personae featured in the social movement narratives analyzed

	Pre-illness		Peri- and post-illness	
	Mainstream	Environmental	Mainstream	Feminist
Villain	The faulty gene Irresponsible risky subject	Corporate and governmental structures that allow exposure to cancerogenic pollutants	Heredity/nature Individuals and organizations not supporting funding for research	Corporate and governmental structures that exacerbate inequalities of access to cancer care
Victim	Risky subject	Collective at risk of the disease	Individuals affected by the disease	Collective affected by the disease
Hero	Previvor	Transdisciplinary research	Survivor Docile biological citizen	Empowered collective

188 HEROES, VILLAINS, AND VICTIMS

chapter. As demonstrated throughout our analysis, social movement narratives around breast cancer have been instrumental in shaping the experiences of women living with or at risk of breast cancer, as well as the modes of funding and researching the disease. There are some notable differences in terms of characterization between the various movement narratives as highlighted in Table 7.1. We further discuss these differences and their effects. For clarity, we will refer to the narratives around the survivorship and previvorship movements as mainstream narratives and those around the environmental and feminist movements as alternative narratives.

5.1 The Plotting of the Central Characters and Their Emotional Appeal

While mainstream narratives center the plot around the heroes (the "previvor" and the "survivor"), the alternative narratives focus on fleshing out a detailed account of the experiences of people living with breast cancer and their struggles. These plotting strategies have important implications for the emotional charge of the narratives.

On the one hand, mainstream narratives' emotional registers revolve around the binary of fear and hope. At the stage of pre-illness, the domain of fear is constructed around the quantification and objectification of risk. In this case, the "previvor" represents the heroic figure of hope who controls her fate by engaging with biomedical rationalities of prevention. At the stages of peri- and post-illness, the domain of fear is constructed around the narratives of war against the disease. In this instance, the domain of hope materializes around (1) the hope for a cure, which is yet to come and requires a generation of funding, and (2) the central character of the narrative, who is the "survivor"—a heroic figure of hope who won the battle against cancer. The emotional binary fear–hope serves as a disciplining tool and a mechanism of social control, which outlines the rights and duties of the biological citizen.

On the other hand, alternative narratives' emotional registers are centered around anger. The anger results from witnessing the experiences of these women affected and/or at risk by breast cancer and their various struggles: struggle in dealing with the disease, struggle to access information and/or care, struggle of their bodies being controlled and judged, and so on. As Polletta (2002) argues, stories provoking emotions of disgust or anger can successfully lead to increasing commitment and mobilizing collective action. In this case, the anger is directed towards the corporate and governmental structures that are responsible for (1) allowing the exposure to cancerogenic pollutants, and (2) exacerbating the inequalities of access to cancer care. Thus, the appeal to emotion in social movement narratives around breast cancer not only contributes to mobilizing collective action but also functions as a disciplining tool for the biological citizen.

5.2 The Characterization of the Villain

While the villain is constructed as a complex character in alternative narratives, its mainstream counterpart is rather simplified. Indeed, the alternative narratives highlight the complexities of the causality of breast cancer and incriminate multiple actors in the process: the alternative narratives refocus the story of causality onto the cancerogenic pollutants, as well as the political, economic, and social structures responsible for not only allowing the exposure to the causal agent but also exacerbating the inequalities of access to cancer care. On the other hand, mainstream narratives rely primarily on the usual biomedical script of cancer as a disease occasioned by the self.

This characterization serves as an essential plot device for the construction of the solution to the problem in each narrative, thereby shaping the modes through which collective action is mobilized. The characterization of the villain, in alternative narratives, draws on multiple sources of knowledge. Similarly to the causal explanation (and subsequently the character), the solution is complex. It involves (1) transdisciplinary research models which include a broader spectrum of disciplines and actors in the understanding of the epidemiology of breast cancer, (2) development of embodied, situated knowledge of the experiences of the different groups of women at risk and/or affected by breast cancer (in particular minority groups), and (3) holding accountable the corporate and governmental structures that are responsible for allowing the exposure to cancerogenic pollutants, and exacerbating the inequalities of access to cancer care. Overall, the solution is framed around the hope for a transformational vision that will shape the breast cancer environment.

On the other hand, the characterization of the villain in the mainstream narratives derives its explanatory power from biomedical rationalities and returns to biomedical rationalities for a solution. In the stage of pre-illness, this solution is represented in the form of wider genetic testing and preventive procedures. In the stages of peri- and post-illness, it materializes in the search for a cure. In order to achieve these aims, there is a need for (1) the compliance

190 HEROES, VILLAINS, AND VICTIMS

of the biological citizen to biomedical rationalities, and (2) the compassion of
the biological citizen in supporting the generation of funding for biomedical
research to find a cure. While hardly visible in the mainstream narratives,
pharmaceutical and biotech companies hold an important role in this process.
As discussed in Section 3, breast cancer is a lucrative disease and holds a firm
top spot in terms of research and development investment and pipeline size.
Indeed, the hope for a cure is a powerful device in generating research funding.
As described by Hopkins and colleagues (2007, 21), the claims underpinning
the biotechnology revolution to attract funding are "rhetorical devices
employed to generate the necessary, political, social and financial capital to
allow perceived promise to emerge."

As for the emotional appeal, this plot device has important implications for
social movement narratives around breast cancer in not only mobilizing
collective action but also as a disciplining tool for the biological citizen. In
addition, the complexity of characterization of the villain can demand additional cognitive effort from the audience to make sense of the narrative, but
also affects how emotions are mobilized. As Fine (2002, 244) argues, the
"cognitive component of stories—their analytical structure—allows audiences
to generalize from their emotions to the worldview that the narrator is
promoting implicitly or explicitly and to make explicit the boundaries that
are otherwise implicit through the placements of heroes and villains in the
narratives."

5.3 The Individualization/Collectivization Dynamics

The movement narratives explored in this chapter highlight different, and
sometimes antagonist, individualization and collectivization dynamics. On the
one hand, the mainstream movement narrative puts the onus on the individual, despite encompassing universalized identity categories (the survivor and
the previvor). On the other hand, the alternative movement narratives create a
collective of a diverse range of individual experiences of being at risk of and/or
living with breast cancer.

While the identity categories of the survivor and the previvor are universalized and the survivorship narrative is collective, the social movement narratives surrounding these characters put the onus back onto the individual. They
do so through the recourse to two devices: the narrative of the responsible
biological citizen and the hopeful configuration of the narrative of breast
cancer activism. First, the mainstream social movement narratives exacerbate

the construction of breast cancer as a disease occasioned by the self. Framing breast cancer as a disease occasioned by the self has important implications for determining the sites of responsibility and blame, which in turn favors the legitimization of particular tools of control that are deemed appropriate to target the source of blame—i.e. the self in this case. While destabilizing the control of the body by conceptualizing a part of it as defective, genetics discourse fosters a sense of control simultaneously, by making additional options available to reduce uncertainty. Thus, genetic information is constructed as empowering individuals through the catering of new choices for health risk management (Hallowell and Lawton 2002). Health risk management becomes an individual moral responsibility, and failing to comply with the ethical practices to "fix" the body and control the risk is, therefore, constructed as moral negligence (Lupton 1995). This process of destabilization has various implications, including the characterization of the various actors within the associated social movement narratives. More than ever, the individual takes center stage with the multiple role of "victim," "hero," and "villain" through embodying the characters "risky subject," "empowered risky subject," and "irresponsible risky subject," respectively.

Second, the usage of positive messages and metaphors in breast cancer narratives can have important implications for the collectivization/individualization dynamics of the mainstream movement narrative. First of all, and as King (2004) argues, an overly optimistic and hopeful configuration of breast cancer has an effect on diminishing the rage of activists particularly with regards to the activism against environmental contaminants, leaving a hereditary/individualist view dominant. Second, the narrative of survivors can alienate women who are going through the side effects of breast cancer treatments, a poor prognosis, or dying from breast cancer (Kaiser 2008). As much as they can be inspiring and uplifting, success stories do not work for everybody, especially for people going through the disease. Their primary function is more geared towards the celebration of the advances and heroism of biomedical sciences, as well as the different actors involved in making the success story a reality. As Ehrenreich (2001, 48) put it: "In the overwhelmingly Darwinian culture that has grown up around breast cancer, martyrs count for little; it is the 'survivors' who merit constant honor and acclaim. They, after all, offer living proof that expensive and painful treatments may in some cases actually work." Finally, the survivorship discourse reconfigures activists' actions through a consumer culture lens (for example, through pushing for the consumption of pink ribbon-branded products as a sign of compassion). Such reconfiguration contributes to reinforcing the processes of individualization, through attaching responsibilities of consumption to the biological citizen. The individualized tone of this movement narrative both reproduces and is complicit in reinforcing the individualization trends in healthcare (Geiger, this volume)—particularly in the realm of geneticized illnesses (Weiner et al. 2017). The fight is performed through individual acts of hopeful and "positive" consumption, rather than collective rage.

On the other hand, the alternative movement narratives put forward a collective narrative of breast cancer etiology and experience. As discussed in our analysis, these narratives are concerned with the representation of the ugly realities of the experiences of women at risk and/or living with breast cancer. The narratives create a space for representing a variety of representations of the embodiment of breast cancer, including those of non-conformist and marginalized identities. By doing so, alternative movement narratives around breast cancer create a collective out of the diverse individual experiences they represent.

As demonstrated throughout our analysis, alternative movement narratives propose an ideological repositioning of the very conceptualization of "risk" when discussing breast cancer. This repositioning has important effects on shifting the epidemiological narrative of breast cancer from a sole focus on the individual to include collective concerns. It is important to note that this shift does not deny or reduce the significance of the embodied experience of being at risk of breast cancer, such as the genetic risk linked to carrying a "faulty" BRCA gene. However, it expands and challenges this view to shed light on alternative scenarios and conceptualizations of risky bodies, as well as the possible entwinement between "faulty" nature and man-made pollutants. Thus, alternative movement narratives contribute to reframing breast cancer etiology as a public health concern rather than a set of personal risk-management strategies promoted and supported by various corporate market actors, such as those focused solely on diet, exercise, genetic screening, and so on.

Furthermore, the ideological repositioning performed by alternative movement narratives has some further implications for the perfect "docile" biological citizen. This persona is morphed into a collective of citizens who mobilize their knowledge and expertise as activists. This new collective entity comes into being with the hope to produce embodied, situated knowledge that can shape our causal understanding of breast cancer, promote alternative modes of prevention, and contribute to policy formulation.

Note

1. It is interesting to note how certain prominent industry actors, such as pharmaceuticals and biotech companies, disappear behind the collective "we"—despite being highly interested parties!

References

Annas, G. (1997), Reframing the Debate on Health Care Reform by Replacing Our Metaphors, in John Glasser and Ronald Hamel (eds) *Three Realms of Managed Care: Societal, Institutional, Individual* (67–75), Sheed and Ward.

Anonymous (1993), You Can't Look Away Anymore, *New York Times Magazine*, September 5. Available at: http://www.nytimes.com/1993/09/05/magazine/l-you-can-t-look-away-anymore-049693.html?mcubz=1.

Bakhtin, M. (1973), Problems of Dostoevsky's Poetics, trans. R. W. Rotsel, Ardis.

Beckmann, N. (2013), Responding to Medical Crises: AIDS Treatment, Responsibilisation and the Logic of Choice, *Anthropology and Medicine*, 20:2, 160–74.

Belkin, L. (1996), How Breast Cancer Became This Year's Hot Charity, *New York Times Magazine*, December 22, 40–6, 55–6.

Bell, K. (2014), The Breast-Cancer-ization of Cancer Survivorship: Implications for Experiences of the Disease. *Social Science and Medicine*, 110, 56–63.

Benford, R. D., and Snow, D. A. (2000), Framing Processes and Social Movements: An Overview and Assessment, *Annual Review of Sociology*, 26, 611–39.

Billig, M. (2008), The Language of Critical Discourse Analysis: The Case of Nominalization, *Discourse and Society*, 19:6, 783–800.

Boje, D. (2001), *Narrative Methods for Organization and Communication Research*, Sage.

Brown, P., Zavestoski, S. M., McCormick, S., Mandelbaum, J., and Luebke, T. (2001), Print Media Coverage of Environmental Causation of Breast Cancer, *Sociology of Health and Illness*, 23:6, 747–75.

Calvès, A. (2009), "Empowerment": généalogie d'un concept clé du discours contemporain sur le développement, *Revue Tiers Monde*, 200:4, 735–49.

CBC News (2013), "Angelina Jolie Effect" Sparks Surge in Genetic Testing: Test Referrals up by 80 Per Cent in Nova Scotia, *CBC News*, October 17. Available at: http://www.cbc.ca/news/canada/nova-scotia/angelina-jolie-effect-sparks-surge-in-genetic-testing-1.2101587.

Centre for Disease Control (2018), What Are the Risk Factors for Breast Cancer? Available at: https://www.cdc.gov/cancer/breast/basic_info/risk_factors.htm.

194 HEROES, VILLAINS, AND VICTIMS

Clarke, J., and Everest, M. (2006), Cancer in the Mass Print Media: Fear, Uncertainty and the Medical Model, *Social Science and Medicine*, 62:10, 2591–600.

Czarniawska, B. (1997), *Narrating the Organisation: Dramas of Institutional Identity*, University of Chicago Press.

Davis, J. E. (2002), Narrative and Social Movements: The Power of Stories, in Joseph Davis (ed.) *Stories of Change: Narrative and Social Movements* (10–34), State University of New York Press.

Derrida, J. (1979), Living on: Borderlines, in Harold Bloom (ed.) *Deconstruction and Criticism* (75–176), London: Continuum.

Desai, S., and Jena, A. (2016), Do Celebrity Endorsements Matter? Observational Study of BRCA Gene Testing and Mastectomy Rates after Angelina Jolie's *New York Times* Editorial, *British Medical Journal*. Available at: http://dx.doi.org/10.1136/bmj.i6357.

DeShazer, M. K., and Helle, A. (2014), Theorising Breast Cancer: Narrative, Politics, Memory, *Tulsa Studies in Women's Literature*, 32–3:2, 7–23.

Edwards, D., and Potter, J. (1993), Language and Causation: A Discursive Action Model of Description and Attribution, *Psychological Review*, 100:1, 23–41.

Ehrenreich, B. (2001), Welcome to Cancerland: A Mammogram Leads to a Cult of Pink Kitsch, *Harper's Magazine*, 43–53.

Evans, G. R., Barwell, J., Eccles, D. M. et al. (2014), The Angelina Jolie Effect: How High Celebrity Profile Can Have a Major Impact on Provision of Cancer Related Services, *Breast Cancer Research*, 16:442. Available at: http://breast-cancer-research.com/content/16/5/442.

Ferraro, S. (1993), You Can't Look Away Anymore: The Anguished Politics of Breast Cancer, *New York Times Magazine*, August 15, 25–27, 58–60.

Fine, G. A. (2002), The Storied Group: Social Movements as "Bundle of Narratives," in Joseph Davis (ed.) *Stories of Change: Narrative and Social Movements* (229–45), State University of New York Press.

Fosket, J. (2010), Breast Cancer Risk as Disease: Biomedicalizing Risk, in A. Clarke, L. Mamo, J. R. Fosket, J. Fishman, and J. Shim (eds) *Biomedicalization: Technoscience Health and Illness in the US* (331–42), Duke University Press.

Fowler, R., Hodge, B., Kress, G., and Trew, T. (1979), *Language and Social Control*, Routledge.

Frank, A. (1995), *The Wounded Storyteller*, University of Chicago Press.

Freire, P. (1974), *Education for Critical Consciousness*, Sheed and Ward.

Gabriel, Y. (2000), *Storytelling in Organisations: Facts, Fictions and Fantasies*, Oxford University Press.

Geiger, S. (2020), Silicon Valley, Disruption, and the End of Uncertainty, *Journal of Cultural Economy*, 13:2, 169–84.

Geiger, S. and Gross, N. (2017), Does Hype Create Irreversibilities? Affective Circulation and Market Investments in Digital Health, *Marketing Theory*, 17:4, 435–54.

Hagan, K. (2013), Breast Cancer: Genetic Testing Soars after Angelina Jolie's Double Mastectomy, *Sydney Morning Herald*, November 13. Available at: http://www.smh.com.au/national/health/breast-cancer-genetic-testing-soars-after-angelina-jolies-double-mastectomy-20131112-2xelm.html.

Hallowell, N., and Lawton, J. (2002), Negotiating Present and Future Selves: Managing the Risk of Hereditary Ovarian Cancer by Prophylactic Surgery, *Health: An Interdisciplinary Journal for the Social Study of Health, Illness and Medicine*, 6:4, 423–43.

Hellomagazine.com 2012. Sharon Osbourne: "Why I Chose to Have a Double Mastectomy," *HELLO!*, November 5. Available at: http://www.hellomagazine.com/celebrities/2012110523415/sharon-osbourne-doule-mastectomy-exclusive/.

Hopkins, M. H., Martin, P. A., Nightingale, P., and Kraft, A. (2007), The Myth of the Biotech Revolution: An Assessment of Technological, Clinical and Organisational Change, *Research Policy*, 36, 566–89.

Hopkinson, G. (2015), How Stories Make It: Antenarrative, Graffiti and Dead Calves, in Michal Izak, Linda Hitchin, and David Anderson (eds) *Untold Stories in Organisations* (285–317), Routledge.

Izak, M. (2014), A Story-in-the-Making: An Intertextual Exploration of a Multivoiced Narrative, *Tamara: Journal of Critical Organization Inquiry*, 12:1, 41–57.

Jacobs, R. N. (2002), The Narrative Integration of Personal and Collective Identity in Social Movements, in Melanie Green, Jeffrey Strange, and Timothy Brock (eds) *Narrative Impact: Social Cognitive and Foundations* (205–28), Psychology Press.

Jolie, A. (2013), My Medical Choice, *New York Times*, May 14. Available at: http://www.nytimes.com/2013/05/14/opinion/my-medical-choice.html.

Jones, Y. (2010), Peeling the Body, PhD Thesis, University of Southampton.

Kaiser, K. (2008), The Meaning of the Survivor Identity for Women with Breast Cancer, *Social Science and Medicine*, 67, 79–87.

Kerr, A., Woods, B., Nettleton, S., and Burrows, R. (2009), Testing for Food Intolerance: New Markets in the Age of Biocapital, *BioSocieties*, 4:1, 3–24.

King, S. (2004), Pink Ribbons Inc: Breast Cancer Activism and the Politics of Philanthropy, *International Journal of Qualitative Studies in Education*, 17:4, 473–92.

King, S. (2006), *Pink Ribbons, Inc: Breast Cancer and the Politics of Philanthropy*, University of Minnesota Press.

Klawiter, M. (2004), Breast Cancer in Two Regimes: The Impact of Social Movements on Illness Experience, *Sociology of Health and Illness*, 26:6, 845–74.

Klawiter, M. (2008), *The Biopolitics of Breast Cancer: Changing Cultures of Disease and Activism*, University of Minnesota Press.

Kolker, E. S. (2004), Framing as a Cultural Resource in Health Social Movements: Funding Activism and the Breast Cancer Movement in the US 1990–1993, *Sociology of Health and Illness*, 26:6, 820–44.

Kushner, R. (1975), *Breast Cancer: A Personal History and an Investigative Report*, Harcourt Brace Jovanovich.

Lorde, A. (1980), *The Cancer Journals*, Spinsters Ink.

Lupton, D. (1995), *The Imperative of Health: Public Health and the Regulated Body*, Sage.

Lupton, D. (2012), *Medicine as Culture*, Sage.

Metzger, D. (1997), *Tree: Essays and Pieces*, North Atlantic Books.

National Cancer Institute, 2015. BRCA1 and BRCA2: Cancer Risk and Genetic Testing. Available at: https://www.cancer.gov/about-cancer/causes-prevention/genetics/brca-fact-sheet.

Olsen, K. A. (2014), Telling Our Stories: Narrative and Framing in the Movement for Same-Sex Marriage, *Social Movement Studies*, 13:2, 248–66.

Osuch, J. R., Silk, K., Price, C., Barlow, J., Miller, K., Hernick, A., and Fonfa, A. (2012), A Historical Perspective on Breast Cancer Activism in the United States: From Education and Support to Partnership in Scientific Research, *Journal of Women's Health*, 21:3, 355–62.

Pal, T., Permuth-Wey, J., Betts, J. et al. (2005), BRCA1 and BRCA2 Mutations Account for a Large Proportion of Ovarian Carcinoma Cases, *Cancer*, 104:12, 2807–16.

Pender, K. (2012), Genetic Subjectivity in Situ: A Rhetorical Reading of Genetic Determinism and Genetic Opportunity in the Biosocial Community of FORCE, *Rhetoric and Public Affairs*, 15:2, 319–49.

Petryna, A. (2004), Biological Citizenship: The Science and Politics of Chernobyl-Exposed Populations, *Osiris*, 19, 250–65.

Pharmaprojects (2019), *Pharma R&D: Annual Review 2019*, Informa.

Polkinghorne, D. (1988), *Narrative Knowing and the Human Sciences*, State University of New York Press.

Polletta, F. (1998), Contending Stories: Narrative in Social Movements, *Qualitative Sociology*, 21:4, 419–46.

Polletta, F. (2002), Plotting Protest: Mobilising Stories in the 1960 Student Sit-Ins, in Joseph Davis (ed.) *Stories of Change: Narrative and Social Movements* (35–56), State University of New York Press.

Potter, J., and Wetherell, M. (1987), *Discourse and Social Psychology: Beyond Attitudes and Behaviour*, Sage.

Potts, L. K. (2004), An Epidemiology of Women's Lives: The Environmental Risk of Breast Cancer, *Critical Public Health*, 14: 2, 122–47.

Rabinow, P. (1992), Artificiality and Enlightenment: From Sociobiology to Biosociality, in Jonathan Crary and Sanford Kwinter (eds) *Incorporations* (234–52), Zone Books.

Rose, N. and Novas, C. (2005), Biological Citizenship, in A. Ong and S. J. Collier (eds) *Global Assemblages: Technology, Politics, and Ethics as Anthropological Problems* (439–63), Blackwell Publishing.

Rothman, K. B. (1998), *Genetic Maps and Human Imagination*, New York: W. W. Norton.

Sharma, A. (2008), *Logics of Empowerment: Development, Gender, and Governance in Neoliberal India*, University of Minnesota Press.

Sigler, H. (1999), *Breast Cancer Journal*, Hudson Hills Press.

Sontag, S. (1978), *Illness as Metaphor*, Farrar, Strauss and Giroux.

Spence, J. (1995), *Cultural Sniping: The Art of Transgression*, Routledge.

Stacey, J. (1997), *Teratologies: A Cultural Study of Cancer*, Routledge.

Steingraber, S. (1997), *Living Downstream: An Ecologist Looks at Cancer and at the Environment*, Addison Wesley.

Sulik, G. (2014), #RETHINKPINK: Moving beyond Breast Cancer Awareness SWS Distinguished Feminist Lecture, *Gender and Society*, 28: 5, 655–78.

Van Leeuwen, T. (1993), Genre and Field in Critical Discourse Analysis: A Synopsis, *Discourse and Society*, 4:2, 193–223.

Weiner, K., Martin, P., Richards, M., and Tutton, R. (2017), Have We Seen the Geneticisation of Society? Expectations and Evidence, *Sociology of Health and Illness*, 39:7, 989–1004.

Willig, C. (2011), Cancer Diagnosis as Discursive Capture: Phenomenological Repercussions of Being Positioned within Dominant Constructions of Cancer, *Social Science and Medicine*, 73, 897–903.

Zavestoski, S., McCormick, S., and Brown, P. (2004), Gender, Embodiment, and Disease: Environmental Breast Cancer Activists' Challenges to Science, the Biomedical Model, and Policy, *Science as Culture*, 13:4, 563–86.

8

The Fantastical Empowered Patient

Samantha D. Gottlieb

Introduction

Renza Scibilia, based in Australia, has an active career as a diabetes patient advocate. On her publicly available blog, *Diabetogenic*, she details the past twenty years living with type 1 diabetes (T1D). Through her blog she describes the advocacy work she has done to address clinicians' language when speaking with or about T1D patients, her push for patient involvement in clinical design and treatment, and her strategies for navigating the emotional and physical demands of a highly demanding chronic disease (Scibilia 2017). During an annual Australasian Diabetes Technologies and Advancements Summit, Scibilia decided to push the mostly clinician audience past their comfort zone, "I knew that there was no way I could talk about the latest diabetes tech advances and not talk about the DIY [do-it-yourself] movement." Using her expertise as both a person with T1D (PWT1D) and her role as a patient educator and advocate, she described the growing movement of open source diabetes technologies. Some clinicians and diabetes technology industry attendees were shocked by the prospect of patient-designed devices, "telling me that I was being irresponsible doing such a thing and even more irresponsible talking about it," but others were curious about the technologies' potential. Scibilia ends with a philosophical proclamation, reflecting on how these tools have impacted her life living with T1D, and how designing her own system offers her a position of power and authority living with a disease that so often requires deference to medical authority.

> I am going beyond simply not following their directions of how I should be managing my diabetes. "You're actually being a deliberately non-compliant diabetic," he [Tim Skinner] said cheekily . . . "This is a lot more than simply being 'non-compliant.' You have actively hacked a diabetes device and are using that to change the way you are managing your diabetes. Deliberately non-compliant!"

Samantha D. Gottlieb, *The Fantastical Empowered Patient* In: *Healthcare Activism: Markets, Morals, and the Collective Good*. Edited by: Susi Geiger, Oxford University Press. © Samantha D. Gottlieb 2021.
DOI: 10.1093/oso/9780198865223.003.0008

He's right. I never thought I'd wear the term 'non-compliant' as a badge of honour, but right then and there, I kind of was.   (Scibilia 2017)

By claiming her use of hacked diabetes medical devices as "deliberately non-compliant," Scibilia challenges clinicians' expectations of what non-compliance means, and she stakes her choice as one that is informed. While she posits this as a "cheeky" (but also quite serious) rebellion/resistance, we might also think of DIY health solutions as uber-compliance. The hyper compliant patients who engage in self-managing their own care by redesigning software and device systems to enhance their lives with T1D. Scibilia's (non) compliance exposes a fundamental tension that PWT1D have long navigated: the clinical expectation that they become experts of their own health and that they demonstrate cooperative deference to medical directives.

T1D is a chronic life-long condition. It occurs when a person's pancreas no longer produces its own insulin. There are more than a million and a half United States (US) residents diagnosed with T1D (American Diabetes Association 2020). T1D requires constant self-monitoring and assessment, as well as reliable and affordable access to insulin, to stay alive. At quarterly endocrinologist visits, patients are evaluated for their "success" at following doctors' recommendations through a blood test that evaluates their past three months of keeping their blood sugar within a prescribed range, known as A1c. If patients have access to the technology of a continuous glucose monitor (CGM), this assessment is supported by data from their medical devices. In 2020, multiple commercial digital platforms exist to customize glucose monitoring and insulin delivery, but as recently as five years ago, these were not yet available. In response to this lack, in the last decade, parents with children who have T1D and PWT1D[1] have designed new methods to live better with diabetes and to reimagine best strategies to manage the disease for themselves or for their children. Not only have they hacked, or reverse engineered, their medical devices, they have disseminated their work through digital open source practices,[2] allowing anyone with access to the proper tools to build their own systems (Leibrand 2014; Lewis 2016, 2017).

Clinical expectations of patients' compliance can encompass a wide variety of criteria, most of which are either subtly or not so subtly about clinicians' authority and power, rather than patients as autonomous individuals. "Compliance" may include (a deliberately incomplete list): participation; following directions; demonstrating a commitment that your doctor knows what's best for you; trusting the ability to achieve the prescribed outcome and the process; belief that the treatment and its potential side effects are better

200 THE FANTASTICAL EMPOWERED PATIENT

than no treatment; believing that one can change one's circumstances and health; having the resources or flexibility in life to implement the changes; having access to the prescribed solutions; and having social support to facilitate your efforts. Yet these imagined evidences of a patient's cooperation fail to account fully for how impossible these standards may be, ignore human complexity, and do not take a patient-centric approach. In short: these expectations and imagined outcomes set many patients up for failure. They offer a clinician-oriented perspective: compliance refers to submission to a voice of authority. As Scibilia implicitly recognizes, non-compliance, then, as a mode of resistance, may be reimagined as a form of patient agency. In this chapter, I consider how some US-based PWT1D reimagine expectations of medical compliance and how their work reveals opportunities for their communities and for patients living with other illnesses to gain agency.

1. Compliance Cast in a New Light: Empowerment

The medical literature that addresses patient compliance assumes that compliance is the appropriate and desirable outcome (Arduser 2017), rather than examining whether patient participation and engagement with their healthcare might take a different cast. Although social scientists have challenged the "rhetoric of compliance" (Segal 2007; Skinner and Franz 2018), clinical health has failed to sufficiently acknowledge how compliance ideology harms patients, the very people clinical health purports to serve. Clinical discourse has gestured toward reframing clinical authority but has yielded only "adherence" as a tepid alternative. I take up Trostle's critique of compliance as ideological, in other words, a conceptual framework and belief system that permeates healthcare in practice and in theory (Trostle 1997, 109). Compliance as ideology highlights compliance's dependency on unequal relationships, such as between doctor and patient.

> [Ideology is] a system of shared beliefs that legitimize particular behavioral norms and values at the same time that they claim and appear to be based in empirical truths. Ideologies help to transform power (potential influence) into authority (legitimate control). *Compliance is an ideology that transforms physicians' theories about the proper behavior of patients into a series of research strategies, research results, and potentially coercive interventions that appear appropriate and that reinforce physicians' authority over health care.* (Trostle 1997, 111, italics added)

Thus, how clinicians deploy compliance in their care for patients may seem abstract, unless one bears the burden of its judgment. In contrast to the prevailing medical literature that seeks to solve how to make patients *more* compliant, I follow Trostle's goal of mapping how compliance defines patient–clinician relationships, and I take it one step further, to sketch out an alternate frame for patient participation, one of agency. I reject the expectation that patients' compliance demonstrates evidence of patients' commitment to their own positive outcomes, and more importantly, I dispute the clinical assumption that what might be called patients' non-compliance indisputably reflects patients' lack concern for their health.

Compliance as a healthcare ideology informs two newer ideological positions that promise to recenter authority in the healthcare setting: patient engagement and (my focus for this chapter) patient empowerment. In the context of diabetes, patients may also be called "activated," to demonstrate their participation in their medical care (Arduser 2017, 18). These are three distinct terms, but they have all crept into medical discourse and US health policy as a promise to reimagine patients' expertise and participation. Although framed as in the best interest of patients, there are more practical (read: economic) reasons that drive the shift. As one website covering digital health trends explains, US healthcare's shift to patient empowerment has ties to the policy push known as Meaningful Use; this policy directive to transition healthcare payments to accountable care organizations sought to increase patient participation in order to drive down US healthcare costs (Dolan 2014). In 2016, the 21st Century Cures Act helped to further the ideological commitment to patient empowerment by requiring the US regulatory agency, the Food and Drug Administration (FDA), to include the patient's perspective in their evaluative criteria (Department of Health and Human Services 2018); as a result, the FDA now assesses the applications of new products with the added requirements of data on patient experiences. These shifts in what constitute data are important; making room for patient narratives allows the regulatory process to account for qualitative and experiential data, but in the implementation of this shift, FDA officials and institutions struggle to make sense of what counts as patient feedback and how pharmaceutical and medical device companies can sufficiently capture evidence of this engagement (Fieldnotes, September 12, 2018). The FDA's codification of patient empowerment in early phases of medical device and pharmaceutical development does not ensure patient-centric approaches throughout the patient's journey and lived experience. Nor does the FDA entirely know how to contextualize the new category of patient data.

202 THE FANTASTICAL EMPOWERED PATIENT

2. Patient Advocacy, Empowerment, and DIY Strategies

The social sciences have identified the emergence of patient-activist-driven empowerment as a strategy of HIV/AIDS activism of the 1980s and breast cancer patient activisms; these two manifestations of patient-led activism reoriented healthcare research to incorporate the patient "expert" and her lived experience (Epstein 1995, 2008). However, as one critique of this literature notes, research on patient-driven activism has disproportionately centered on US breast cancer and HIV/AIDS patient-led activism, framed as "vanguard activist groups" (Petersen et al. 2019, 6). More contemporary exploration of patient-led activism includes identifying how patients gain scientific expertise through their experience managing their health conditions, drawing on daily and embodied practices (Pols 2014, 75). There are many examples of patient activisms that transcend the patient-as-expert model; patient involvement in their medical diagnoses, treatments and related research are diverse and do not always follow historical forms of activism (Klawiter 2002; Callon and Rabeharisoa 2008; Akrich 2010; Pols 2013; Rabeharisoa et al. 2013; Ebeling 2019; see also Rabeharisoa and Doganova, this volume and Cheded and Hopkinson, this volume). Indeed, in some cases, groups joined by shared health status, such as the deaf community, have used their collective efforts to reject technologies designed by outsiders (Blume 1997).

The democratization, technologization, and domestication of medical tools have expanded the methods with which patients can enact "citizen science" (Childerhose and Macdonald 2013; Wiggins and Wilbanks 2019); and indeed, "public participation has lost much of its adversarial edge" and is even now courted by corporations and regulatory entities (Kelty and Panofsky 2014, 2; see also Galasso and Geiger, this volume). Individuals who are not professional scientists or researchers can now build their own experiments, tinkering with their physiologies, collecting data to track their behaviors and to inform behavior or health changes (Callon and Rabeharisoa 2008; Nielsen and Langstrup 2018; Lehtiniemi and Ruckenstein 2019). Modern technologies have accelerated and diversified the ways patients can redesign their healthcare interventions, but independent actors have long been embedded in technoscience practices. Thus, although HIV/AIDS patients' advocacy may have contributed to a shift in patients' roles in the production of scientific knowledge, patients have long been co-contributors to knowledge and expertise.

Design-thinking frameworks and a growing commitment to participatory design in clinical research have gained traction in recent years, in some cases promoting work that citizen scientists have done, allowing for an increase in patient participation in commercial research and development (Delgado et al. 2011; Rowland et al. 2017). Patient-driven innovation or the "right" amount of activism (meaning: not too much) has also found support in clinical and regulatory settings (FDA 2017). The empowered or engaged patient, in these initiatives, is typically turned into an exemplar of specific "[b]iosocial groupings—collectivities formed around a biological conception of a shared identity biological citizenship" (Rose and Novas 2005, 442). Biological citizenship constrains how one can know oneself as an individual, genetic and somatic, and as part of a broader population. Digital technologies have led to new forms of bio-digital citizenship: digital media and technologies facilitate and circumscribe individuals' participation in their health, and patients' advocacy and participation in policy and innovation may take place on digital platforms (Petersen et al. 2019). As Langstrup has suggested, drawing on Althusser's concept of interpellation, patients' involvement in research and design enrolls patients into a particular identity and use of potential technologies: "Interpellation not only makes the subject recognize himself or herself in certain ways but also sets in motion new actions related to and transformative of the logic[s]" (2011, 5). These patient groups presented with the potential of empowerment then "come to feel obliged to respond not only to the promises of cures and therapies but also to the identities that they are promised" (2011, 6).

In this chapter, I demonstrate how the PWT1D movement, juxtaposed against the FDA initiatives to increase patient engagement through an empowerment discourse, highlights how patient interpellations can produce radically different logics of "what it means to be a patient." Patients can and often do present creative approaches to their health, but regulatory frameworks do not account for patients' adaptive critiques of formulaic medical management. These evolving practices of patient participation, research and development for treatments and devices, policy and regulatory interventions, and health condition-specific communities unsettle the boundaries of clinical and institutional health authorities. The rest of this chapter will consider how some PWT1D communities simultaneously exemplify the idealized highly engaged patient *and* the deliberately non-compliant patient, presenting an identity that may seem contradictory or near impossible: the fantastical empowered patient. By calling them fantastical, I call attention to medical discourse's implied impossibility of engaged, non-compliant patients, who are absolutely real, agentic people—as evidenced by the multiple thousands of

204 THE FANTASTICAL EMPOWERED PATIENT

PWT1D who use novel technological strategies to reclaim agency and reimagine their life with diabetes (Lewis 2020).

3. Methods

This chapter draws on anthropological research I conducted between 2015 and 2019. The project initially focused on the PWT1D open source software community who publicly disseminated their technological interventions, such as the DIY Pancreas System/Open Artificial Pancreas System (APS), Nightscout, and Loop, to improve others' experiences living with T1D. As the research evolved, I broadened the focus to capture the larger policy and clinical discourses around open source software in healthcare, patient engagement, and regulatory concerns. This chapter draws on forty-one interviews with individuals (thirty-one) and parents (seven) of children with T1D,[3] endocrinologists (two), and patient advocates (two) for other health conditions. In addition, some of these PWT1D interlocutors lead diabetes-oriented companies or organizations. Ethnographic observations include three FDA workshops, four diabetes conferences, four T1D hackathons (2016–18), Twitter diabetes social media, and one pharmaceutical conference (not focused on diabetes) promoting patients as "partners." I conducted twenty-eight in-depth interviews via video conferencing or telephone, and the rest in person, but there were many additional informal conversations with my interlocutors when we met in person,[4] e.g., at the Hackathons or diabetes conferences, that inform my research. I interviewed one FDA official off the record, and thus cannot quote her, but she enhanced my understanding of some of the questions the FDA has grappled with, as they add patient engagement to their evaluative criteria. All interlocutors' names have been changed in this chapter to respect their anonymity, except in the cases when they spoke to me as public figures or I cite their statements in publicly available documents. This work was aided by a research assistant, who is a PWT1D. Data have been analyzed with computer assisted qualitative data analysis software (Atlas.ti). I analyzed the primary and secondary data with grounded theory and inductive methods. Although I do not have T1D, nor do I have family who are PWT1D, I come to this work as a person living in the US who has been a patient, often disempowered and frustrated by the US healthcare system that consistently invests in the wrong things.

4. Automating the Pancreas

A highly truncated history of the T1D community's path to building their own technologies follows. Fifty years after the first patient received insulin, T1D management tactics remained little changed, but in the past half century, the domestication of tools for T1D have altered the life and management of T1D (Hedgecoe 2002). In the late 1970s and early 1980s, the availability of "self-monitoring" glucose testing allowed patients to test blood glucose levels at home, instead of only at the clinic/hospital. Insulin-dependent people, as all T1D are, inject insulin with syringes or, more recently, with insulin pens or insulin pumps. Insulin pumps, commercially available since the 1980s, are a more discreet method to deliver insulin (Melvin 2016). Originally a backpack-sized device, insulin pumps have gotten much smaller but are still a bulky appendage, worn on a belt or tucked into a pocket, with tubes connecting the pump to the wearer's body. Although modern pumps with tubing are the size of a 2020 smartphone, the tubeless insulin pump worn on the arm, about a quarter of the size of a 2020 smartphone, marketed as OmniPod, first approved by the FDA in 2005, presents yet another insulin-delivery option (FDA 2005).

Diabetes technology has advanced beyond diversifying insulin delivery; advances in sensor technology made the personal CGM possible in 1999 (Olczuk and Priefer 2018). Individuals can now wear a small device, embedded in the skin, to read interstitial fluid that then converts the information into a glucose reading (DiSimone 2019). CGMs have gone from "error machines," as my interlocutors have called them when recalling the earlier incarnations of the technology, to a much more reliable stream of data, updated every five minutes. Instead of having to prick a finger for a traditional glucose meter and then infer whether one's sugar levels are going up or down, or what behavior or food may have impacted the single data point, the CGM generates a dynamic graph for its wearers, with predictive direction for their glucose levels and historical data; the nearly continuous data allow users to interpret better how their bodies respond to different behaviors (such as exercise) or health states (such as menstrual cycles or illness). The CGM can provide users with deeper insights into how their body responds to different life circumstances. Users no longer have to interpret the variables that might be impacting "why...the insulin [is] not doing what it's supposed to be doing" or grappling with "the anger...that came from just not knowing. If you stick your finger at breakfast and you're 100, or whatever, it doesn't even matter, and then you stick your finger at dinner and you're 300 you're just sort of like, 'oh it sucks because I'm 300 now'" (Charlie, thirty-three, T1D twenty-five years). For many, the CGM is a decoder. As Deanne, fifty-six years old, living with T1D for twenty years, who does not use a hacked system, explained,

> It was so eye-opening to be able to look down, see a number, see a trend, see what the food does, have the alerts, because, before, I had a lot of lows ... I'd rather give up a pump than give up my [CGM] because ... the [CGM] to me is lifesaving. Yeah, it tells me where I'm at all the time, where I'm going to go, and it feels like I can go to sleep at night and not wonder [about my glucose levels].

Nearly every interlocutor talked about the CGM as one of the most meaningful devices to manage their diabetes.

In spite of CGM's availability in the early 2000s, it wasn't until 2011 when two hackers identified a security flaw in the leading manufacturer's (Medtronic) insulin pumps, which eventually would allow others to extract data from the insulin pumps and to connect their CGMs to inform pump behavior (DiFranco 2014). Medtronic and other manufacturers designed their pumps with proprietary software, limiting patients' access to the pumps' data. Medtronic required a "CareLink" USB device to extract the pumps' data, and Medtronic further restricted data access to clinicians who had the software to export the data in their office. Patients, the people who lived with diabetes, wore the pumps, and generated the data on the pump, could not freely access their own data. Without manually correlating glucose levels with insulin delivery, it remained difficult to make informed choices about insulin dosages or alter diets or behaviors.

> Originally, you could have one of the meters that they could download at the endo[crinologist] and get all of your numbers off of it, just because writing in the book was a chore. So that was like level one. And then ... we have CGM data, but it's locked in the device.
>
> (Theo, thirty-five, T1D for twenty-five years)

For many living with T1D, they sought data access to interpret their own physiologies.

> I really just wanted CSVs or Excel sheets of my data to do some visualizations on my own, and so I was really looking for tools, but I happened on Ben's GitHub account as well as Dana's blog, and so I started piecing some of that

together on my own and figuring out, okay, it turns out I can probably talk to some other things.   (Charlie, thirty-three, T1D twenty-five years)

Further complicating patients' use of their own data, insulin pumps, such as Medtronic's, were not interoperable with other manufacturers' glucose monitors.

It turns out the software for the Medtronic pump and the software for the Dexcom don't work together, and. . . they don't run on a Mac or a Mac family . . . I started doing some hacking, minor, not serious hacking . . . just fiddling around with browser settings and with emulators to make them run on my Mac. And I finally get it all to work, and I post the instructions on an online user group forum for Medtronic users . . . that forum was run by Medtronic, and they removed my post . . . in 2013, late 2012 . . . if you actually took the time to read . . . some of the privacy policy and user agreements . . . some of them said crazy stuff like, "by using our software or using our service you give up all right, title and interest to the data." And I was like, "Are you kidding me? No. This is my daughter's data, it's her disease. No."

(Luther, Father of T1D adolescent)

Geographically distant and independently, PWT1D struggled to better use the data their pumps generated, data to which they believed they ought to have reliable access.

One individual involved in the early reverse engineering of device software, Ben West, wrote an open letter to the FDA emphasizing the importance of knowing what his devices were doing and having access to the data his body generates. "Many patients are actively harmed by lack of access to epistemic certainty of what to expect from their therapy . . . the fidelity of their care is poor because they are prevented from empirically understanding their own therapy or ensuring its safety" (West 2012). West focused on trust in the devices upon which his life depends and noted that the locked software could cause more harm than good. "Without constant action to manually over-ride the pump, the pump will give me the incorrect amount of insulin, causing insulin reactions and in some cases even contributing to severe hyperglycemia requiring hospitalization" (2012). In other words, West's (and subsequent DIY interventions') alternative approaches to device use allowed individuals to make safer and more appropriate decisions about treating their T1D.

While these efforts could be seen as the disobedient acts of isolated individuals, a more cohesive patient movement soon emerged, bringing together disparate individuals who shared a commitment to data as a key component of living with T1D. Those who decided to hack the software found each other through online and offline communities. Online communities, like "CGM in the Cloud," a Facebook group for those seeking to share their data with family and caregivers, provided a resource for families. Eventually, a group of individuals formed a non-profit organization, Nightscout, run by PWT1D families (Nightscout 2015). Nightscout adopted the hashtag #WeAreNotWaiting (a phrase coined by a PWT1D parent who works in the diabetes industry during a diabetes conference run by a T1D individual who is a diabetes consultant and has ties to a number of corporate entities).[5] The ability to see their T1D children's data remotely reduced parents' stress and worry they experience daily, yet commercial entities continued to drag their feet on this technological development. Nearly all my interlocutors had heard clinicians promise a cure for T1D was only five years away, even though for some PWT1D the five-year-promise is now more than forty years old. #WeAreNotWaiting reflects the community's distrust in diabetes-related corporations and the technologies available (Best 2012; Arduser 2018; Nightscout 2018). The hashtag makes explicit the reclamation of autonomy over their (and their children's) care. Not only does the hashtag reflect a refusal to wait for the asymptotically-always-five-years-away diabetes "cure," it now includes the bricolage and hacking of medical devices (both software and hardware) to create the tools to improve life with the chronic disease (Lewis 2014a, 2017). The DIY movement does not ask permission to engage from regulators or commercial entities, it asserts it. The DIY movement is not empowerment externally conferred upon patients; the communities have reimagined their agency.

As diabetes technologies advanced, the various communities (not all online) began to focus their efforts to bridge the connections between CGMs and insulin pumps. A number of individuals, including Dana Lewis and her partner Scott Leibrand, were able to design a system that Lewis and Leibrand called the DIY Pancreas System in 2013. The system initially focused on adjusting alarms on Lewis' CGM, which at the time were not loud enough to wake her up during hypoglycemic events. Ben West independently had designed some of the early interfaces between the devices, and over time a number of other individuals contributed to the Open APS through online collaborations posted on GitHub.[6] In 2014, Lewis experienced her first day "looping," as it is called when the CGM and insulin pump form a closed feedback loop. As she posted on her blog, "the outcomes are awesome. In fact, they are better than I expected!" (Lewis 2014b). Around the same time, Nate Rackleyft, collaborating with Chris Hanneman and Pete Schwamb, developed an iOS system, known as Loop (Rackleyft 2016). The DIY systems available now work on diverse software platforms and are highly customizable to meet the various needs of different kinds of users and caregivers.

The open source T1D community has challenged the siloed and proprietary systems of diabetes medical devices, building algorithmic systems that allow the CGM to affect the pump's behavior. The burden of constant calculations, oversleeping important nighttime alarms, basal level doses that don't account for hormonal, or nighttime, or exercise variations, have been technologically outsourced and semi-automated to make it easier for people who are already living with the anxieties and uncertainties that diabetes introduces into their lives. These hacks and the perseverance of those engaging in them are impressive; equally importantly, the community has taken the work they've put into the systems they've created (Loop, Open APS, Open Android) and shared it online, so that, in theory, anyone can build their own system—and in doing so created a DIY patient movement. The open source philosophy and the community-oriented nature of their work makes it possible for people to learn from others and to benefit from the changes that individuals have achieved for their own families. Accessing out-of-warranty pumps or necessary supplies to support these devices depends on a grey market distribution; this not only benefits the community at large, as the sharing of older devices brings more people in to support the project, but it also represents the community's direct challenge to existing models of healthcare. They connect the digital, the material, and the social into an effective and impactful change in their communities' lives.

> It was insanely empowering to look at this thing that I've never done before and I mean, really it's like copying and pasting somebody else's code but you never know. Shit can go wrong. It can *not* work…I felt very empowered and…look, I can do this.   (Sydney, forty-five, T1D for thirty-seven years)

As Sydney describes, she draws upon the labor of others who have helped to develop the systems, but she downplays how much effort and wherewithal it requires for a person to circumvent existing structures and institutionalized barriers to a different (individualized, responsive) management of diabetes. Although Sydney calls it empowerment, what she describes might be better termed agency and autonomy.

The medical device revolutions fomented by T1D communities demonstrate the power of what it means to truly allow patients to lay claim to their own tools and to assert their expertise. The open source DIY T1D movement offers a real-world example of how hypothetical patient empowerment *can* and *does* actually happen. But the community's efforts also reveal the limitations in the empowerment discourse: institutional calls for patient participation assert defined boundaries and do not offer the same opportunities to patients whose conditions are less data-dependent or who may not have as much daily self-management. Finally, although the PWT1D communities who have designed and built their own systems are exceptionally motivated and effective, their efforts do not solve the many inequities in T1D disease management, especially in the US. Open source solutions have yet to solve the high cost of insulin[7] and the uneven access to T1D technologies (DiFranco 2014; Madley 2019; Pear 2019; Smith 2019). Although this chapter does not focus on these significant disparities among communities of PWT1D, these issues of access and cost lurk as problems that must be solved through policy and regulatory interventions rather than patients incurring the burden of "empowerment" to solve a problem that individuals cannot directly impact. As the communities I worked with acknowledge, the DIY open source movement is only part of the solution to improving the quality of life for PWT1D.

4.1 The Food and Drug Administration and the Promise of Empowerment

During the same period that PWT1D open source communities have redesigned their medical devices, software, and disease management strategies, the US FDA has concurrently emphasized patient-centric expectations for its regulatory standards (FDA 2017; Rao 2017). In the last five years, the FDA and its Centers for Device and Radiological Health (CDRH, pronounced "cedar"), which regulate medical devices, have focused on mechanisms to increase patient empowerment or "engagement" (FDA 2017). Language choices matter, as members of the PWT1D, and other communities living with disabilities, remind the public. Regulatory and commercial definitions of patient involvement have real impact on the everyday lives of those living with chronic disease. The PWT1D tactics and strategies, which reconfigure institutional ideas of patient involvement, contrast notably with the FDA's efforts to increase patient involvement in health research, development, and regulatory processes.

Indeed, even the FDA's Patient Engagement Advisory Committee (PEAC), formed in 2017, does not accord patients a participant role, but only an advisory one. At one PEAC meeting I attended, the chair, Paul Conway, explicitly articulated its review of the FDA's plan for "Connected and Empowered Patients: e-Platforms Potentially Expanding the Definition of Scientific Evidence...to better engage patients and consumers as empowered partners in the work of protecting public health and promoting responsible innovation" (FDA 2018). In this meeting, it became clear how the slippage between "empowerment" and "engagement" further constrains patients' limited agency. Claims of empowerment and engagement suggest patients have the power (and authority) to be agentic individuals, but in practice (and particularly in relation to the national regulatory body, the FDA), this rarely is true.

In the last five years, the FDA has reimagined the patient role in medical product development and regulation. In late 2015, the FDA created PEAC to grapple with the shifts in healthcare practice and to surface patient concerns. As they announced in their *FDA Voice* newsletter:

> We are entering an era of "patient-centered" medicine in which patients and their care partners participate actively in decision-making and priority-setting about all aspects of health care. Americans are becoming increasingly active consumers of health care, making choices about their doctors, diagnostics, treatments, and healthcare experiences rather than simply allowing health care providers to make the decisions for them...While it's important to consider patient perspectives, we understand that patients still expect FDA to do our primary job—namely, ensuring the safety and effectiveness of FDA- regulated medical devices.   (Hunter and Califf 2015)

As part of this larger push within the FDA, CDRH has facilitated workshops and advisory committees for the patient voice, including 2017 and 2018 PEAC meetings (open to the public) and a variety of other patient engagement-oriented workshops. The 21st Century CURES Act, passed in the US Congress in 2016, requires clinical trial data to include "Patient Reported Outcomes" and "Patient Preference Information" to acknowledge and to incorporate experiences and data that have traditionally fallen out of the standard clinical trial endpoints. The emphasis is on earlier stage regulatory and clinical trial development stage, and this likely has little impact on clinician–patient interactions.

At one 2018 CDRH conference I attended in Baltimore, Maryland, "Medical Devices–Patient Engagement in Real World Evidence," the FDA officials repeatedly asked how to turn "data into evidence" and what to do with, what they called, qualitative data's "anecdotes." Despite the expectation to

212   THE FANTASTICAL EMPOWERED PATIENT

bring evaluation categories that included patient-generated data into their regulatory evaluations, these perspectives remain a "problem" due to their presumed variability and complexities that evaluative structures have yet to integrate. As they parsed the implications of potential ambiguities, they undermined the premise of the event—that patients offer valuable and essential insight into medical device experiences. These worries, I would argue, are ill-founded, as the T1D open source movement has demonstrated. Patient needs are not a hodge-podge. They are coherent and well founded. At the conference, officials asked me and a sociologist, who happened to be attending for fieldwork too, about these perceived limits of qualitative data, as though there were not more than forty years of medical anthropology, medical sociology, and science and technology studies to give contour to their questions. One program manager detailed the FDA's position on how to structure data, insistent that qualitative data lack the necessary replicability to be useful for the FDA. At the 2018 conference, FDA officials worried whether qualitative data could be sufficiently generalizable and struggled with what they feared could be unstructured patient-collected data. At its heart, however, the distrust of "qualitative" or experiential data emphasized the institutional skepticism with patient-driven data.

No one raised the question of whether quantitative clinical data might also have their ambiguities or whether the assumptions in quantitative data could also be messy and problematic. Nor did they sufficiently recognize that qualitative data *can* be structured. Even more troubling, they did not ask about how existing data categories might efface patient insights. During the group break-out session, I suggested that quantitative data have their limitations, too, and although some FDA officials nodded in assent, they ultimately asserted quantitative data were a gold standard; the question already settled that this was the proper way to organize knowledge. The officials sought to give credence to patient expertise, but they disavowed its value by treating it as noise, rather than a meaningful signal. Throughout the sessions, it struck me how starkly the FDA strategies to incorporate patients juxtaposed with the strategies the DIY T1D community had deployed. The FDA-driven shift to patient empowerment purports to recast power to patients' hands, but even in this framing, the FDA bestows power by conceding its evaluative structure might benefit from patient wisdom. Empowerment does not come through patients' resistance, but rather it is permitted by those in positions of authority. A CDRH FDA official explained to me a couple of months later, off the record, that the agency has yet to solve the tension of truly encouraging innovation that comes in non-traditional forms or facilitating patients to become advocates who can assist building better models, such as the work achieved by the DIY T1D community. In other words, the DIY T1D model, which exemplifies what empowerment might look like, unsteadies the institutional conceptions of innovation or empowerment.

The T1D communities have leveraged a key strategy of engaging, as the founder of Tidepool, Howard Look, puts it in public talks, "early and often" with the FDA. This approach has thus far protected the PWT1D projects and has allowed them to avoid being shut down by regulatory censure. After years of building and disseminating open source systems, the first FDA warning came in April 2019 after an individual using a hacked system had an adverse event (FDA 2019). As many, including Dana Lewis and Ben West, point out, the DIY systems that they're using "fail" back to the standard settings of the insulin pump. In other words, the risk of the system is no more dangerous than the danger of living with a pump (FDA approved) and living with T1D (a significant risk to all PWT1D). A non-functioning DIY system is the system that endocrinologists prescribe all the time and to which the FDA has accorded regulatory approval.

Risk and safety are recurring themes for both critics and advocates of the DIY strategies. Proponents of DIY systems remind critics that living with diabetes is intrinsically risky. Too much insulin can kill you. Diabetes-related health complications can be very serious. Living with T1D, regardless of medical tools, means living with a high risk of long-term diabetes-related morbidities and risk of death. Social systems, such as schools and workplaces, do not sufficiently support living with an invisible disability and thus present "risky" spaces. The DIY APS options allow for families and communities to navigate these structural failures with remote and digital forms of care, which mitigate these risks. Were there to be more direct FDA challenges to the DIY systems, they would be directly calling into question the very products that have received regulatory approval.

4.2 Empowerment Does Not Always Mean Agency

So here she is, the fantastical empowered patient. She has found a resource that perhaps many other PWT1D do not have. She has tapped into the community of PWT1D using open source-distributed guidance documents to build her own T1D system. The PWT1D open source communities have brought together the FDA-approved devices and paired them to semi-automate their daily tasks. For most people using the systems, these tools have led to better control, more predictable outcomes, and overall better quality of life, by reducing the time thinking about diabetes incessantly. It is not a casual endeavor. It is a superlative amount of engagement with one's health. The subset of this community, those who have written the code and developed the algorithms or those who use the openly shared code to build their own systems, could not better fit into the empowered patient paradigm. And yet, their deliberate actions do not match these imagined empowered patients that the FDA have sought to incorporate into their models. As those tinkering with their systems have learned, even the empowered/compliant patient can be thwarted from being permitted control over her tools.

Despite new labels and allusions to alternate models of patient participation, discourses of empowerment and engagement in healthcare resemble long-existing compliance discourses. Patients living with chronic disease who refuse to follow the compliance ideology risk stigma and censure or even the inability to access the care they need. In the U.S., patients' failure to "comply" may lead to doctors writing notes in patient records that in turn may impact health insurance payments or clinicians' willingness to treat them. Even as patient empowerment promises to recenter the patient in her healthcare, the distinct imaginaries of the empowered patient's involvement in her healthcare, offered by the FDA or pharmaceutical industries, do not facilitate patients' agency. Hugo Campos (2015), a vocal patient advocate who figured out how to access the data on his implanted pacemaker, explained it to me as autonomy: "I will do whatever it takes to regain my autonomy, to regain my ability, my right to self-determination. That's very strong in me." As Campos navigated the loss of insurance, which in turn meant the loss of monitoring for his hypertrophic cardiomyopathy, he discovered how disempowered he really was. "Their philosophy to this day is that the doctors have all the knowledge, the patients are supposed to be compliant, and that's not . . . I don't agree with that." Campos, like many in the T1D communities, decided to circumvent regulations, insurance obstacles, and gatekeeping of information management, in order to live more safely with better insight into the tools that help to keep him alive.

The role of the empowered patient requires enlisting a particular set of resources, energies, and collaborations in order to receive treatment as a whole person. As Tracy, an interlocutor who runs a patient advocacy organization for a non-T1D health condition, told me, even active and engaged patient participation does not always lead to the care a person needs, "you go in there because you need help. If you're being kicked out because you're empowered, you're not getting help." Empowerment, much like compliance, is a prescriptive and ideological category, dependent on a specific power distribution in the patient–clinician relationship. Tracy and Renza Scibilia remind us that there are implicit limits to patient empowerment. Their participation and disruption of traditional patient–clinician roles provoke the question: *when* does the patient transform from being engaged to becoming problematic? For many with whom I spoke, their disruptions of established practices are not deliberate forms of activism, but rather individuals seeking support and finding the structures and resources lacking. People like Hugo Campos, who used self-education to learn how to extract data from his pacemaker, can only push the movement so far. Exceptions, like Hugo or Tracy, show what lengths individuals must go to for self-advocacy, and how the transition of their efforts to a collective movement is an overwhelming, and perhaps unattainable, process.

Lest the T1D DIY projects be a tale of techno-triumph, we must recognize that although the DIY tools promise a form of liberation, my interlocutors remind me that they still live with diabetes, with the possibility of technology failures, and a slew of unpredictabilities that cannot be fully automated or eliminated.

> There's too many variables and, like, yeah, software makes it better but it still has to get into my body ... And to continue to generate your own ability to live, agency, pleasure, health. Yeah. I think that's the thing. Like the self as the generation source rather than a technology as a generator.
>
> (Sophia, thirty-two, T1D for twenty-seven years)

Just as the deliberately non-compliant actor may feel empowered and agentic, there are, as in all parts of life, many places where one cannot control outcomes perfectly. Sensors detach, allergic reactions to adhesive tape happen, tubes get damaged, or the wearer forgets to turn the system back on after a shower. Regardless of technology access, however, a fundamental challenge for people who are insulin-dependent in the US is that insulin remains nearly unaffordable to many. The open source DIY PWT1D communities recognize the multiple variables that might fail or cause harm, but they choose a path that allows them to make the distinctions between which risks to take and which are too much to bear. For them, as it should be for most patients, this is the path of agency.

Many of my interlocutors have questioned the term patient directly, wanting to reject the implications of its constraints, its relationship to power, expertise, and authority. One interlocutor, Janet, positions herself as a consumer, which presents a vast set of assumptions and economies to trouble, even as her proclamation emphasized new possibilities.

216   THE FANTASTICAL EMPOWERED PATIENT

> You can buy a cell phone today for your mom. You can also buy a cell phone for your teenager, they're pretty much 180-degree ends of the spectrum. Why aren't medical products that way? It's because we don't think about medical products with consumers in mind we think of patients, and patients are captive.   (Janet, fifty-four, T1D for thirty-nine years)

In her version, the consumer holds the power and implies the freedom to choose alternate options. "I have made myself a consumer. You can see very clearly, I'm not a patient. I'm not a patient in any sense of the traditional word or not, but I have made myself a consumer, and I've been really successful" (Janet). Most of the T1D hackers and creators, some of whom would not call themselves advocates, do not want the task of advocate or empowered patient, on top of the demands of living with a chronic disease; however, the health industry celebrates the empowered patient positionality,[8] easily commodifiable, as though such beneficence were the path to corporate compassion. Empowerment thus becomes an empty and false mantel.

Conclusion

The fantastical empowered patient is fantastical because the person must exist in a nexus of time, resources, and savvy, as well as being seen and heard as a fully embodied patient in the clinical setting that is available to too few. Private commercial decisions, as Ruha Benjamin reminds us in the context of racism latent in technology, are still public policy decisions (2019, 12). The T1D open source communities that have accomplished so much are predominantly white, middle- and upper-middle-class, highly educated people. Carl, who self-identifies as an African-American PWT1D, sees it as his mission to increase representation among digital communities and across diabetes types, "It's already a known fact that diabetes affects people of color more than non-people of color, so it makes no sense that there shouldn't be more people of color involved in it ... There needs to be more representation" (Carl, fifty-five, T1D for thirty years). These communities' diverse pursuits of access to technologies and tools are a form of entitlement that all patients should, but unfortunately do not, have. They believe they should have access to treatments, that they should be able to ask the questions about the treatment they receive, and to feel able to resist what is offered. We should all feel entitled to do this in the context of our healthcare. In the T1D hackers' deliberate pushbacks against top-down notions of patient empowerment and in their pursuit of their own versions of agency, they are rare and inspiring, but they also call attention to their exceptionalism. Despite the intention of universality and accessibility in the deliberate choice of open source strategies, there are many visible and invisible barriers to DIY-ing one's own diabetes care, and thus, we must question this as a sustainable strategy. The diverse communities of PWT1D need alternatives that recognize variability, specificity, and alternatives to the existing model of care.

This exceptionalism requires acknowledging an absence in Scibilia's creative reclamation of others' judgment of her actions. As with other reclaimed epithets, how ought a deliberately non-compliant patient protect against being read as the "accidental/non-deliberate non-compliant" T1D? Deliberately non-compliant exists in a binary—if "deliberate non-compliance" is an intentional position that those who embrace it see as informed and well defended, then do those who are non-deliberately non-compliant (or, just regular people for whom the bar for "compliance" is unachievable) remain a problem? This question holds true for empowerment, too, reminding us how these purportedly novel terms perpetuate the very dynamic that Scibilia and others want to reimagine.

What constitutes appropriate engagement if we preserve the terms, even jauntily, that designate a power differential? While Scibilia's deliberate stance challenges the clinical categorizations of "problematic" T1D behavior, it does not sufficiently protect those who cannot, or do not wish to, comply from censure in the clinical context. The open source T1D community is thus fantastically empowered because they operate on a different plane, not just within the constraints of typical clinical–patient relationship. They neither reject medical knowledge, nor do they propose specious solutions to their frustrations. They work within the system but offer a radical alternative. What remains unclear is how well regulatory and commercial research and development structures will ever fully account for their innovation, both within the diabetes space and in other chronic health conditions. The open source DIY T1D accomplishments are a story of patient agency, rather than "empowerment." As the DIY PWT1D have made unambiguously clear, agency can and does radically change patient lives—and seeking it, therefore, is an activist undertaking.

Acknowledgments

This work was funded by a National Science Foundation grant, SES-1632716. I am grateful for the generosity of my interlocutors, who have shared their lives and their struggles with

218 THE FANTASTICAL EMPOWERED PATIENT

me. Jonathan Cluck contributed to the research and offered invaluable insights into the research that informed this work. During the revision phase of this research, I was employed by Fitbit, which has since been acquired by Google, Inc., however all research and the writing of this chapter were conducted while I was an independent scholar. This project was motivated by the incessant exhaustion that chronic health patients experience navigating the US healthcare system. We all deserve better.

Notes

1. Some individuals living with T1D prefer the term "diabetic," while others prefer to be called "people with T1D." For this chapter, I have chosen the latter term, putting people, not the disease, first. I use it interchangeably for parents whose children have T1D and individuals managing their own T1D. These are distinct communities, however, with discrete concerns, but their shared concern for access to data and management have led to shared contestations of T1D technology.
2. The free/open source software movements occupy a complex political economy, but open source is not only a software philosophy (Coleman 2013); health and science research has had its moments valorizing public accessibility, for example, Frederick Banting's decision to sell the patent for insulin to the University of Toronto in 1921 for $1 (roughly the equivalent of $14 in 2019).
3. In one instance, an interlocutor is both a parent of a child living with T1D and a PWT1D. Two of the parent interviews were conducted with parent dyads who manage their child's T1D.
4. Fourteen of the remotely conducted interviews were interlocutors I met or interacted with in person during the course of research.
5. I lack space to discuss this here, but many of the individuals pushing forward DIY interventions or challenging the status quo are also embedded in the diabetes medical device or medical education industries. This makes them distinct from other disease health advocates who may not have the familiarity with competing business concerns nor have access to networks of decision makers.
6. GitHub is a repository for software projects that allows users to duplicate and change projects that they might not be able to "write" over. It is a centralized location for software code that allows disparate users to share.
7. As Carl, a fifty-five-year-old PWT1D told me, "one of the things that unifies people with diabetes, no matter what religion, political affiliation . . . They relate to not being able to pay 500 dollars for a bottle of insulin or, having to ask for help."
8. In the last five years, industry-related conferences focusing on patient participation have proliferated, including one I attended called "Patients as Partners" (https://theconferenceforum.org/conferences/patients-as-partners/2019-recap/). These conferences tend to downplay industry ties, even as all the sessions are led or include corporate employees. There is also a diabetes-related event that happens twice a year, framed as a patient-led event (as it is organized by a PWT1D), but it, too, has deep ties to commercial interests. Attendance is by invite only, and it is difficult to find online information about it, although social media are a useful resource. I have attended three

of these conferences and presented a talk at one of them with my research assistant. I received no compensation for participation and since it occurred within driving distance did not receive any coverage for expenses, but I did not pay registration fees and was allowed to eat the food served at the event.

References

American Diabetes Association (2020), Statistics about Diabetes. Available at: https://www.diabetes.org/resources/statistics/statistics-about-diabetes.

Akrich, Madeleine (2010), From Communities of Practice to Epistemic Communities: Health Mobilizations on the Internet, *Sociological Research Online*, 15:2, 10.

Arduser, Lora (2017), *Living Chronic: Agency and Expertise in the Rhetoric of Diabetes*, Ohio State University Press.

Arduser, Lora (2018), Impatient Patients: A DIY Usability Approach in Diabetes Wearable Technologies, *Communication Design Quarterly Review*, 5:4, 31–9.

Benjamin, Ruha (2019), *Race after Technology: Abolitionist Tools for the New Jim Code*, John Wiley & Sons.

Best, Rachel Kahn (2012), Disease Politics and Medical Research Funding: Three Ways Advocacy Shapes Policy, *American Sociological Review*, 77:5, 780–803.

Blume, Stuart S. (1997), The Rhetoric and Counter-Rhetoric of a "Bionic" Technology, *Science, Technology and Human Values*, 22:1, 31–56.

Callon, Michel and Rabeharisoa, Vololona (2008), The Growing Engagement of Emergent Concerned Groups in Political and Economic Life Lessons from the French Association of Neuromuscular Disease Patients, *Science, Technology and Human Values*, 33:2, 230–61.

Campos, H. (2015), The Heart of the Matter. Available at: http://www.slate.com/articles/technology/future_tense/2015/03/patients_should_be_allowed_to_access_data_generated_by_implanted_devices.html.

Childerhose, J. E., and Macdonald, M. E. (2013), Health Consumption as Work: The Home Pregnancy Test as a Domesticated Health Tool, *Social Science and Medicine*, 86, 1–8.

Coleman, E. G. (2013), *Coding Freedom: The Ethics and Aesthetics of Hacking*, Princeton University Press.

Delgado, Ana, Lein Kjølberg, Kamilla, and Wickson, Fern (2011), Public Engagement Coming of Age: From Theory to Practice in STS Encounters with Nanotechnology, *Public Understanding of Science*, 20:6, 826–45.

Department of Health and Human Services (2018), Docket No. FDA–2018–N–4000, Framework for a Real-World Evidence Program; Availability, *Federal Register*, 83:235, December 7.

220 THE FANTASTICAL EMPOWERED PATIENT

DiFranco, A. (2014), Superseding Institutions in Science and Medicine, *BioCoder*, Winter, 23–34.

DiSimone, K. (2019), FDA Warning against DIY Systems, May 20. Available at: http://seemycgm.com/2019/05/20/fda-warning-against-diy-systems/.

Dolan, B. (2014), In-Depth: A Brief History of Digital Patient Engagement Tools, February 21. Available at: https://www.mobihealthnews.com/29985/in-depth-a-brief-history-of-digital-patient-engagement-tools.

Ebeling, M. F. (2019), Patient Disempowerment through the Commercial Access to Digital Health Records, *Health (London)*, 23:4, 385–400.

Epstein, Steven (1995), The Construction of Lay Expertise: AIDS Activism and the Forging of Credibility in the Reform of Clinical Trials, *Science, Technology and Human Values*, 20:4, 408–37.

Epstein, Steven (2008), Patient Groups and Health Movements, in Judy Wajcman, Michael Lynch, and Olga Amsterdamska (eds) *The Handbook of Science and Technology Studies*, MIT Press.

FDA (2005), 501 (k) Premarket Notification for Insulet Insulin Pump, January 3. Available at: https://www.accessdata.fda.gov/scripts/cdrh/cfdocs/cfpmn/pmn.cfm?ID=K042792.

FDA (2017), Enhancing FDA's Approach to Patient Engagement: Current State Analysis and Recommendations, May. Available at: https://www.fda.gov/media/109891/download.

FDA (2018), Public Workshop—Fostering Digital Health Innovation: Developing the Software Precertification Program, September 12. Available at: https://www.fda.gov/medical-devices/workshops-conferences-medical-devices/public-workshop-fostering-digital-health-innovation-developing-software-precertification-program.

FDA (2018), Patient Engagement Advisory Committee, Center for Devices and Radiological Health Medical Devices Advisory Committee. Transcript, November 15. Available at: https://www.fda.gov/advisory-committees/advisory-committee-calendar/november-15-2018-patient-engagement-advisory-committee-meeting-announcement-11152018-11152018.

FDA (2019), FDA Warns People with Diabetes and Health Care Providers against the Use of Devices for Diabetes Management Not Authorized for Sale in the United States: FDA Safety Communication, May 17. Available at: https://www.fda.gov/medical-devices/safety-communications/fda-warns-people-diabetes-and-health-care-providers-against-use-devices-diabetes-management-not.

Fieldnotes from Medical Devices and Patient Engagement Workshop, Baltimore, MD September 12, 2018.

Hedgecoe, Adam M. (2002), Reinventing Diabetes: Classification, Division and the Geneticization of Disease, *New Genetics and Society*, 21:1, 7–27.

Hunter, Nina L., and Califf, Robert M. (2015), FDA Announces First-Ever Patient Engagement Advisory Committee, *FDA Voice*.

Kelty, C., and Panofsky, A. (2014), Disentangling Public Participation in Science and Biomedicine, *Genome Med*, 6:1, 8.

Klawiter, Maren (2002), Risk, Prevention and the Breast Cancer Continuum: The NCI, the FDA, Health Activism and the Pharmaceutical Industry, *History and Technology*, 18:4, 309–53.

Langstrup, Henriette (2011), Interpellating Patients as Users: Patient Associations and the Project-Ness of Stem Cell Research, *Science, Technology, and Human Values*, 36:4, 573–94.

Lehtiniemi, Tuukka, and Minna Ruckenstein (2019), The Social Imaginaries of Data Activism, *Big Data and Society*, 6:1, 205395171882114.

Leibrand, S. (2014), A DIY Artificial Pancreas System? Are We Crazy? February 7. Available at: https://diyps.org/2014/02/07/a-diy-artificial-pancreas-system/.

Lewis, D. (2014a), What Is #DIYPS (Do-It-Yourself Pancreas System)? June 20. Available at: https://diyps.org/2014/06/20/what-is-diyps-do-it-yourself-pancreas-system/.

Lewis, D. (2014b), How Does a Closed Loop Artificial Pancreas Work When You DIY? Or: #DIYPS Closed Loop Is Working! December 15. Available at: https://diyps.org/2014/12/15/how-does-a-closed-loop-artificial-pancreas-work-when-you-diy-or-diyps-closed-loop-is-working/.

Lewis, D. (2016), Live Interview with Dana Lewis, Creator of Do-It-Yourself Pancreas System (#DIYPS), *TuDiabetes*, January 13. Available at: https://tudiabetes.org/event/live-interview-with-dana-lewis/.

Lewis, D. (2017), Next Generation #OpenAPS Hardware Work in Progress—Pi HATs, October 22. Available at: https://diyps.org/2017/10/22/next-generation-openaps-hardware-work-in-progress-pi-hats/.

Lewis, D. (2020), OpenAPS Outcomes, July 13. Available at: https://openaps.org/outcomes/.

Madley, Rachel (2019), Does Anyone Really "Love" Private Health Insurance? *New York Times*, September 17, sec. A, p. 23.

Melvin, A. (2016), The Evolution of T1D Technology, October 26. Available at: https://beyondtype1.org/the-evolution-of-diabetes-technology/.

Nielsen, Karen Dam, and Langstrup, Henriette (2018), Tactics of Material Participation: How Patients Shape Their Engagement through E-health, *Social Studies of Science*, 48:2, 259–82.

Nightscout (2015), What Is the Nightscout Project? Available at: http://www.nightscout.info/.

Nightscout (2018), For the Times They Are A-Changin, June 25. Available at: https://www.nightscoutfoundation.org/news/2018/6/25/for-the-times-they-are-a-changin.

Olczuk, D., and Priefer, R. (2018), A History of Continuous Glucose Monitors (CGMs) in Self-Monitoring of Diabetes Mellitus, *Diabetes Metab Syndr*, 12:2, 181–7.

Pear, Robert (2019), Lawmakers in Both Parties Vow to Rein in Insulin Costs, *New York Times*, April 10, sec. A, p. 17.

Petersen, Alan, Schermuly, Allegra Clare, and Anderson, Alison (2019), The Shifting Politics of Patient Activism: From Bio-sociality to Bio-digital Citizenship', *Health: An Interdisciplinary Journal for the Social Study of Health, Illness and Medicine*, 23:4, 478–94.

Pols, Jeannette (2013), The Patient 2.Many: About Diseases That Remain and the Different Forms of Knowledge to Live with Them, *Science and Technology Studies*, 2, 80–97.

Pols, Jeannette (2014), Knowing Patients, *Science, Technology, and Human Values*, 39:1, 73–97.

Rabeharisoa, Vololona, Moreira, Tiago, and Akrich, Madeleine (2013), Evidence-Based Activism: Patients' Organisations, Users' and Activists' Groups in Knowledge Society, *CSI Working Papers Series 033*.

Rackleyft, Nate (2016), The History of Loop and LoopKit, October 2. Available at: https://medium.com/@loudnate/the-history-of-loop-and-loopkit-59b3caf13805.

Rao, N. (2017), The FDA's Mirror Moment: Will a New Office Reflect Patients' Needs? Available at: https://whatsthefix.info/fdas-mirror-moment-will-new-office-reflect-patients-needs.

Rose, Nikolas, and Novas, Carlos (2005), Biological Citizenship, *Global Assemblages: Technology, Politics, and Ethics as Anthropological Problems*, Wiley, 439–63.

Rowland, P., McMillan, S., McGillicuddy, P., and Richards, J. (2017), What Is "the Patient Perspective" in Patient Engagement Programs? Implicit Logics and Parallels to Feminist Theories, *Health (London)*, 21:1, 76–92.

Scibilia, R. (2017), Deliberately Non-Compliant Diabetic, October 25. Available at: https://diabetogenic.wordpress.com/2017/10/25/deliberately-non-compliant-diabetic/.

Segal, J. (2007), From "Compliance" to "Concordance": A Critical View, *Journal of Medical Humanities*, 28:81–96.

Skinner, D., and Franz, B. (2018), From Patients to Populations: Rhetorical Considerations for a Post-Compliance Medicine, *Rhetoric of Health and Medicine*, 1:3–4, 239–68.

Skinner, Tim (@Tims_Pants), "I take issue with the abstract that #WeAreNotWaiting users are 'reprogramming their devices.' Quite the opposite. We are using existing communication protocols to allow external systems to program them according to manufacturer guidelines, to use them more effectively." Tweet, September 16, 2019, 8:09.

Smith, Dana G. (2019), Biohackers with Diabetes Are Making Their Own Insulin, *Elemental*, May 30. Available at: https://elemental.medium.com/biohackers-with-diabetes-are-making-their-own-insulin-edbfbea8386d.

Trostle, James A (1997), The History and Meaning of Patient Compliance as an Ideology, *Handbook of Health Behavior Research II*, Springer, 109–24.

West, B. (2012), Letter to FDA's Helene Clayton-Jeter. Insulaudit: Hacking Diabetes: Open Source Driver to Audit Medical Devices, June 21. Available at: https://github.com/bewest/insulaudit/blob/master/questions/eff.markdown.

Wiggins, A., and Wilbanks, J. (2019), The Rise of Citizen Science in Health and Biomedical Research, *American Journal of Bioethics*, 19:8, 3–14.

9

Markets, Morals, and the Collective Good after Covid-19

Barbara Prainsack and Hendrik Wagenaar

When reading the very rich contributions to this edited volume, we could not help thinking: How has the current crisis changed all this? How has the Covid-19 crisis affected the configuration of social, economic, and political factors that underpin the practices we are analyzing in our work? This hesitation, of course, is not a reflection on the robustness of the analyses presented and the conclusions drawn in the eight preceding chapters. It results from our own confusion about what the pandemic has changed, and what is still "the same." If anything, the Covid-19 crisis has shaken up some of the things we considered practically immutable; it has shattered Big Truths—such as that we "cannot afford" more social protection—and smaller ones, such as that white-collar work needs to take place in an office. The crisis has changed what we consider doable and thinkable.

We believe it has also changed our moral landscapes. Let us take solidarity, a term that is often evoked in the current crisis. If we understand solidarity, as we do in our work (Prainsack and Buyx 2011, 2017), as practices by which people support others with whom they feel they have something in common,[1] then solidarity has been rather volatile since the beginning of the pandemic. Many people feel that after an initial surge in the beginning of the Covid-19 crisis, solidarity has tapered off. People have lost their enthusiasm to go out of their way for others, especially if these others infringe their own sense of safety and security. Many people just can no longer see those who behave differently than they do as part of the bigger "We." Because of the high stakes of the crisis, differences in how we deal with it have begun to define who we are. Irritations and conflicts over what we perceive as risky behavior create barriers that obstruct the view on what connects us. In Austria, our own country of residence, representative surveys show that the proportion of people who agree that "we're all giving our best to overcome the crisis," "most people agree that mutual support is important," and "we're working together to

Barbara Prainsack and Hendrik Wagenaar, *Markets, Morals, and the Collective Good after Covid-19* In: *Healthcare Activism: Markets, Morals, and the Collective Good.* Edited by: Susi Geiger, Oxford University Press. © Barbara Prainsack and Hendrik Wagenaar 2021. DOI: 10.1093/oso/9780198865223.003.0009 protect the most vulnerable" has decreased continuously in the first year of the crisis (Prainsack et al. 2020; see also Kittel et al. 2020).

But this person-to-person solidarity is, of course, not the only type of solidarity there is. One of us, in her earlier work (Prainsack and Buyx 2011, 2017), proposed to differentiate between interpersonal, person-to-person solidarity (tier 1), solidarity at the group level (tier 2), and solidarity crystallized in legal, administrative, and contractual norms and institutions (tier 3). This third, institutionalized form of solidarity has anything but tapered off during the crisis. People who used to scream "nanny state" and turn away in disgust at even the slightest attempt to affirm or expand the public sector, are now calling for well-funded public healthcare systems, or demand more effective social security measures (e.g. Downie 2020). It has become apparent that countries with stable and well-funded solidaristic institutions are better prepared to weather many aspects of the crisis than those countries that do not. Their citizens are less prone to losing their incomes and homes, and their overall health status is better. Even social unrest is less pronounced in countries with lower levels of social inequalities (United Nations Development Programme 2019). What the Covid-19 crisis has made clear so far is that investments in social services and public infrastructures "pay off." The costs of crises are lower when collective responsibility—manifested in public services and infrastructures organized according to the principle of solidarity (i.e. access based on need, contributions based on ability to contribute)—is higher. In sum, while interpersonal solidarity has fluctuated during the first year of the pandemic— the type of person-to-person solidarity that manifests itself in running errands for vulnerable neighbors or refraining from going out to protect strangers— the importance of institutionalized solidarity has increased (Prainsack 2020).

Does this mean that the larger moral landscape has shifted? We believe that it has. It has shifted in a way that also affects the role of markets. First of all, against the backdrop of what we have learned in the Covid-19 pandemic so far, it seems to become increasingly clear that people are better off if they need not satisfy their fundamental needs on "the market." Fundamental needs (rather than wants) are the basic requirements to survive, to participate in society, and to live with a modicum of security and dignity. Some of these needs—such as food or clothing—can be satisfied by things that people can buy. Others—such as healthcare, elder and childcare, housing, transport, education, and information—cannot. They should be provided publicly. This does not mean that we should return to the "good old age" of the centralized provision of exclusively state-run services. Proponents of the movement for Universal Basic Services (UBS) in the United Kingdom, for example, seek to "overhaul the traditional model of public services so that they are genuinely participative, controlled by the people who need and use them, and supported rather than always directly provided by the state" (Coote and Percy 2020, 5). The main role of the state, then, would be to provide the legal framework within which these services will be provided, and to prescribe and monitor standards—while the provision of the services should work through cooperatives, citizen initiatives, and private vendors.[2]

As we argue in our book *The Pandemic Within: Policy Making for a Better Society* (Wagenaar and Prainsack 2021), it is hard, against this backdrop, to retain the narrative of government being the ineffective, slow, and somewhat thick little sister of private enterprise, characterized by ingenuity, flexibility, and innovation. And indeed, commercial digital enterprises—ranging from education technology to videoconferencing and online shopping platforms to telemedicine—have adapted, improved, and scaled their products at a breath-taking pace. But as the Covid-19 crisis has also shown, where societies have relied on commercial competition to satisfy other, more basic needs such as healthcare, housing, or merely the provision of protective equipment, things did not go so well. For for-profit enterprises, driven by the imperative of maximizing shareholder value, preparing for the remote eventuality of a pandemic that may or may not take place in the future is not a viable business strategy. The United States even saw the ironic situation that private hospitals, deprived of routine check-ups and interventions as their income source, had to hope that new infections would rise as they would then be eligible for public emergency funding at least (e.g. Khullar et al. 2020). At the same time, when vaccines against Covid-19 became available at the end of 2020, many state bureaucracies failed in getting them to the people fast enough, at the cost of human lives. This is, in part, a result of failing political leadership and defective public administration, the latter brought about by decades of bleeding out the public sector, to which we will return below. Resources—including human resources—for human health had been cut in many countries also in the public sector (for an argument of how this matters in the Covid-19 crisis, see Harford 2020). Moreover, when being a public servant is no longer a cause for pride, but a sign that one is seemingly not good enough to get a "real" job in the private sector, it is no wonder that those who can run off to better paid and more prestigious jobs in the corporate sector. But still, even in this situation, governments in many countries have reacted in a fast, flexible, and innovative manner. They have thrown a lot of money at the crisis, money that has prevented even more people from losing their jobs, homes, and livelihoods.

So, where does the idea of the inherent deficiencies of the public sector come from? In the 1960s, James Buchanan, an economist from the University of Virginia, published a series of books in which he presented an economics of government.[3] "Public choice economics," as the movement was called, was supposed to create "useful tools for analysing the incentive structures of public life" and "nonmarket decision-making" (Maclean 2017, 79, 85), which essentially meant the systematic introduction of business accounting and other rationalities and metrics into the analysis of public administration. This was based on the assumption that in politics, just as in regular markets, rationality and self-interest are closely linked. Political actors such as politicians, voters, interest groups, and bureaucrats, so Buchanan and his followers assumed, were subject to the same self-interested, utility-maximizing behavior as the buyers and sellers in the commercial markets for fashion or consumer electronics. And because bureaucrats in particular, so Buchanan argued, held an information advantage over the political leadership in terms of the "goods" they produced, they could extract a surplus from their political superiors. Thus, government agencies intrinsically produce a larger output than is actually needed or required (Niskanen 1971), leading to an ever greater expansion of government. This was the "scientific" proof of what many conservatives in leading positions in business, academia, and politics had suspected all along: government had metastasized to the point that it stifled the market and ruined public finance.

Public choice economics set out to put an end to this. Armed with its main instruments of deregulation, privatization, shrinking the state, and stimulating the market, it became a growing movement also on other continents. In Europe, it came in handy as a tool for Margaret Thatcher's offensive against the welfare state (MacLean 2017, 83). But public choice had developed within a data-free environment and most of its assumptions, when put to the test, proved to be empirically wrong. Bureaucrats were not always keen on expanding their agency, especially not when it meant taking tasks on board that did not fit their mission (Wilson 1989). Salaries of bureau chiefs were not proportionate to bureau size. Political leaders could regularly rely on much more information than public choice theorists had claimed. It was impossible to say at what point public agencies produced excessive outputs of public goods, just as it is difficult to determine the value of such goods (Self 1993, 34). In fact, public choice theory was not a theory at all but a doctrine, an ideology, deliberately clad in the garments of science (Maclean 2017, 80). Its aim was to shield private property from the federal government, defend the freedom of corporations, and limit the functions of the state to those of the libertarian night watchman state: defense against external and internal enemies, upholding and adjudicating property laws, and fending off threats to the optimal functioning of the free market (Gamble 1994). In the words of historian Nancy Maclean: "In the movement's view, government was the realm of coercion, and the market was the realm of freedom, of freely chosen, mutually valued exchange" (2017, 208). Funded by wealthy corporate backers, public choice advocates sought to attain their ends by limiting taxation and shifting tax burdens to lower-income groups, suppressing voting, restricting or even outlawing unions, deregulating corporations and financial institutions, curtailing social protection programs and state-subsidized healthcare, privatizing education and pensions, and changing the constitution to lock in these changes (Maclean 2017, xvii; see also Pistor 2020).

Via tools such as New Public Management, the ideology of public choice economics spread over large parts of the world (e.g. Kettl 2006). Because capitalism took specific forms in different parts of the world, creating particular environments for government and public administration (Hall and Soskice 2001), the proliferation of public sector management practices was uneven. But its ideational component, a deep distrust of the state and the constraint of the autonomy of public administrators, created, ironically, the fulfillment of its own prophecy: that "the state" was ineffective, paper-heavy, slow, and dusty. If you need to get something done, including in healthcare, leave it to a private enterprise. Right?

Scholars such as Mariana Mazzucato have done a great deal to debunk the myth of private enterprise as the sole engine of innovation (Mazzucato 2015). As she and others have shown, public funding of basic research, as well as public services and infrastructures such as education, transportation, and financial instruments secured and protected by state regulation, are the real enabler of technological innovation. This has also become apparent in the development of Covid-19 vaccinations. But emphasizing that the state can do technological innovation just as well as private businesses leaves two important things unsaid. First, Kean Birch and colleagues recently warned against the uncritical celebration of technological innovation, arguing that in recent decades, a good part of technological innovation has created little or no value in the real economy. Instead, it often amounted to another form of rent seeking (Birch et al. 2020; see also Birch 2017a, 2017b). The legal protection of intellectual property (IP) is a case in point: it has shifted from the IP itself to protecting the financial investments into IP assets (Birch et al. 2020). This means, in turn, that it is no longer society at large, or the most vulnerable people in it, that benefit from it, but the economically most powerful, such as investors and shareholders. Birch and colleagues conclude that, rather than a solution to contemporary global challenges, "innovation" may lie at the root of these problems. This is another important aspect of markets and morals: Whom does technological innovation serve, and at whose costs? In societies that are characterized by ever greater social and economic inequalities, it is no longer good enough to talk about the collective good; instead of claiming that something does, or does not, serve the collective good or the public interest, we need careful scrutiny of how different groups within our collective are affected differently. This does not imply a retreat from the notion of a collective, or the idea that there is such a thing as a collective good. It is a commitment to serving people within the collective in equitable ways.

This brings us to the second point that Mazzucato and her followers leave out of their otherwise helpful analyses. While they emphasize the role of the "entrepreneurial state" as a technological innovator, they do not say much about the state as a social innovator. But it is on this front that "the state" has achieved some of its most impressive results. As Hendrik Wagenaar and Florian Wenninger showed in a recent article about "Red Vienna," the state can be, and has been, both a visionary and architect of social change (Wagenaar and Wenninger, 2020). Red Vienna is the name of a period of enlightened public administration in the Austrian capital between 1919 and 1933. In the space of a mere fourteen years, facing, upon its installation, the economic, infrastructural, and human devastation of World War I, the social democratic city administration designed and implemented a large-scale integrated program for housing, public health, education, health, and cultural policy that has withstood the test of time. More than a century later, Vienna is still seen as the world capital of public housing (Förster and Menking 2018), with presently over half the population living in social or other publicly funded or subsidized housing—without the stigma that is attached to public housing in other countries, and often in high-quality buildings in pleasant leafy neighborhoods or in the city center.[4] At the heart of the remarkable success of Red Vienna was a body of well-trained civil servants endowed with a clear administrative ethos, creative and progressive tax policies, a pragmatic approach towards experimentation, the institutionalization of solutions that worked, and a progressive humanist vision of improving the physical, mental, and educational condition of the working class. The government of Red Vienna returned values of fairness, justice, equality, and aesthetics to government (see also Wagenaar and Prainsack, 2021, chapter 4). And while Red Vienna came to a bitter end with the rise of Austrofascism, in postwar Europe, the state—in the form of courageous political leaders, crafty administrators, and visionary civil society and interest organizations—continued their path of social innovation. Poverty was alleviated or even averted due to codification of workers' rights, social security, and universal healthcare. In the 1970s, educational and welfare reforms made higher education available to groups who had not had access previously, and increased social mobility. Solidaristic practices that had been in the making since the late 1900s were expanded and combined into comprehensive, universal welfare state arrangements that improved security and dignity especially for the disadvantaged and marginalized. Sadly, two or three generations have now grown up, who, under the influence of the anti-state, anti-government ideology that we described above, cannot imagine the state as a force for the good. And even if they could, they believe that the money is not available for the state to provide a social infrastructure for all.

During the Covid-19 crisis it has become clear that the market-oriented ideology of the minimal state has left governments ill prepared to weather the pandemic and its economic and social effects. As is apparent in our empirical studies on how people in Austria fare within the Covid crisis (Kieslich et al. 2020; Kittel et al. 2020), many do not want to return to the old normal. Instead, they want less consumption, a more sustainable economic system, and fewer working hours (which should not be confused with "working less"—productivity does not, of course, decrease or increase proportionally with the hours worked). All of this is closely related to improved physical and psychological health and well-being. For many people, health has obtained a new meaning. They have experienced first-hand how important it is to have well-funded and high-quality healthcare that is accessible for all—and they have experienced how much of our health is not shaped by healthcare but by other factors: social protection, safe and stable housing, social contact, access to green spaces, and a job that pays a living wage and does not make you sick.

But how do we get there? The current political-economic constellation does not provide much reason for optimism. The Covid-19 crisis has revealed major problems with business and with government. In many countries, governments are overwhelmed, political polarization has increased, fueled by social media (and sometimes stoked by opportunistic political leaders), and large businesses see the crisis as an opportunity to increase their power and wealth. Although we need action on the side of government and business to get out of this mess, we cannot expect them to do this on their own. The liberal democratic model that has governed the advanced economies of the West has reached its limit. Its economic and social externalities have caught up with it. It is in need of serious reform.

The outline of such reform would combine the legitimacy of democratic influence, the effectiveness of expert administration, and the openness and creativity of associational life within civil society. It would apply these principles to all realms of public life. Differently put, it would break down the firewall between economy and society that is characteristic of our current landscape of markets, morals, and the collective good. We need to enlarge the scope of democratic influence. Issues that are central to human flourishing, such as work and money, need to be brought under democratic control. In general, economic transactions need to be treated as an intrinsic part of social and natural life, subject to their customs and requirements, and not a separate domain opposite and in many instances antithetical to social life.

We envision a model of government that rests on three principles: a rich associational civil society, problem-driven practical deliberation, and the creation of intermediary structures that mediate between state agencies and associational civic life. Civil society associations and initiatives are incubators of creative solutions, they teach people democratic skills, they are pragmatic and problem-oriented, and they fulfill an important monitor function. They hold governments and businesses to account and pressure them to act on unacceptable social ills and urgent problems. They influence the political agenda. But civil society associations are too fragmented and too local to do this on their own. They lack the resources, such as money and political influence, to realize their values and ideas. Moreover, many of our most pressing problems (that all impact people's health), such as climate change, extreme income inequality, and violent conflict, operate on higher levels of aggregation. For this reason, we need intermediary structures to connect the creative and transformative power of citizens and their associations to the decision-making power of the state. This is not an easy task, but there are historical and contemporary examples that attempted to do just that. They may serve as inspiration for contemporary solutions of institutional transformation. But difficult or not, a closer union of civil society and the state, collaborating as equals, is our only alternative. In other words, more societal and economic domains that are now operating according to the principles of competition, growth, and efficiency need to be characterized by institutions of solidarity. Thus, health activism in the post-Covid-19 world should aim for increasing meaningful participation of all stakeholders, including patients, family members, and caregivers, in decisions on how healthcare should be provided. But it also requires a push for adequate funding for healthcare that is accessible to all. It means considering health in all domains of policy and practice (see e.g. Puska 2007), in participatory ways, and committed to the reduction of inequities. Turning care—for the ill, elderly, and the very young— into a collective responsibility and a publicly provided service according to the principle of solidarity forms the normative foundation of the much needed institutional shift.

Again, this does not mean a return to exclusively state-provided and centralized planning and service provision—but it does require a reconsideration of the role of the state. The state needs to become a promotor and steward of the collective good again, and not primarily a protector of business interests and promotor of austerity. The role of data is one of the golden threads throughout this volume. Such a new health and care activism does not seek to devalue data-driven practices. Whereas trends facilitated by digital practices such as personalization and precision (see especially the chapters by Geiger, Galasso and Geiger, Moran and Mountford, and Hoeyer and Langstrup, in this volume), with their focus on big data, individualization, and, to some extent competition, embody some developments that work against the idea of collective benefit (see also Dickenson 2013), they could also be used for the sake of personal and collective wellbeing. Data collected at the individual level do not need to be used solely for the benefit of the same individual, or a corporation seeking to profit financially from the data. The data could also be used to promote public health and collective wellbeing—for example, by using data to learn where public services should be concentrated because they would meet the greatest need; or where public infrastructures should be improved (Rasmussen et al. 2020).

For this strategy to work, however, we need to change how we frame public policy problems. When obesity is framed as a correlate of stress and deprivation, then the answer will be to improve social protection, workers' rights, and affordable housing; if it is framed as a lack of individual self-control, the answer will be nudging. Similarly, when public policy problems are framed in such a way that they are attentive to the structural factors and social determinants that represent their root causes, then the responsibility to solve these problems will be on collectives, on public authorities and communities. This is also an element of health and care activism within the new moral landscape in the post-Covid-19 world. It will be the collective task of citizens, politicians, and other decision makers to focus on the collective side of health and care within the new moral landscape in the post-Covid-19 world.

Notes

1. These commonalities are not "objectively" existing characteristics that people merely recognize in a factual way. Instead, these commonalities are recognized (or not) according to the ways in which people have learned to structure social and political space. They are the categories of othering dominant in our societies, and in our own communities.

2. The British UBS initiative covers services in the context of shelter, food, health, education, transport, information, and the legal and democratic domain (see also universalbasicservices.org). In a typical Organisation for Economic Co-operation and Development country, the provision of UBS is estimated to amount to around 4.3 percent of gross domestic product (Coote and Percy 2020, 115).
3. For a more detailed history of the grand narrative of government failure, see Wagenaar and Prainsack (2021).
4. This is not to say that Vienna hasn't seen its share of deregulation and rent increases; we describe these in Chapter 4 in Wagenaar and Prainsack (2021).

References

Birch, K. (2017a), Rethinking Value in the Bio-economy: Finance, Assetization and the Management of Value, *Science, Technology and Human Values*, 42:3, 460–90.

Birch, K. (2017b), Financing Technoscience: Finance, Assetization and Rentiership, in D. Tyfield, R. Lave, S. Randalls, and C. Thorpe (eds) *The Routledge Handbook of the Political Economy of Science* (169–81), Routledge.

Birch, K., Chiappetta, M., and Artyushina, A. (2020), The Problem of Innovation in Technoscientific Capitalism: Data Rentiership and the Policy Implications of Turning Personal Digital Data into a Private Asset, *Policy Studies*, 41:5, 468–87.

Coote, A., and Percy, A. (2020), *The Case for Universal Basic Services*, Polity Press.

Dickenson, D. (2013), *Me Medicine vs. We Medicine: Reclaiming Biotechnology for the Common Good*, Columbia University Press.

Downie, J. (2020), The Pandemic Has Turned Conservatives into Their Liberal Boogeymen, *Washington Post*, May 10. Available at: https://www.washingtonpost.com/opinions/2020/05/10/pandemic-has-turned-conservatives-into-their-liberal-boogeymen/.

Förster, W., and Menking, W. (eds) (2018), *The Vienna Model 2: Housing for the City of the 21st Century*, Berlin: Jovis.

Gamble, A. (1994), *The Free Economy and the Strong State: The Politics of Thatcherism*, Basingstoke: Macmillan.

Hall, P. A., and Soskice, D. (2001), An Introduction into Varieties of Capitalism, in P. A. Hall and D. Soskice (eds) *Varieties of Capitalism: The Institutional Foundations of Comparative Advantage*, Oxford University Press, 1–71.

Harford, T. (2020), Why We Fail to Prepare for Disasters, *The Financial Times*, April 16. Available at: https://www.ft.com/content/74e5f04a-7df1-11ea-82f6-150830b3b99a.

Kettl, D. F. (2006), *The Global Public Management Revolution: A Report on the Transformation of Governance*, Brookings Institution Press.

Khullar, D., Bond, A. M., and Schpero, W. L. (2020), Covid-19 and the Financial Health of US Hospitals, *JAMA*, 323:21, 2127–8.

Kieslich, K., El-Sayed, S., Haddad, C. et al. (2020), From New Forms of Community to Fatigue: How the Discourse about the Covid-19 Crisis Has Changed, November 12, Blog post. Available at: https://digigov.univie.ac.at/solidarity-in-times-of-a-pandemic-solpan/solpan-blog-english/blog-posts/news/from-new-forms-of-community-to-fatigue-how-the-discourse-about-the-covid-19-crisis-has-changed-1/?tx_news_pi1%5Bcontroller%5D=News&tx_news_pi1%5Baction%5D=detail&cHash=8a5c34534be62ffe5c578d6721435eeb.

Kittel, Bernhard, Kritzinger, Sylvia, Boomgaarden, Hajo et al. (2020), The Austrian Corona Panel Project: Monitoring Individual and Societal Dynamics amidst the Covid-19 Crisis, *European Political Science*. Available at: https://doi.org/10.1057/s41304-020-00294-7.

Maclean, N. (2017), *Democracy in Chains: The Deep History of the Radical Right's Stealth Plan for America*, Scribe.

Mazzucato, M. (2015), *The Entrepreneurial State: Debunking Public vs. Private Sector Myths*, Anthem Press.

Niskanen, W. A. (1971), *Bureaucracy and Representative Government*, Aldine Atherton.

Pistor, K. (2020), *The Code of Capital: How the Law Creates Wealth and Inequality*, Princeton University Press.

Prainsack, B. (2020), Solidarity in Times of Pandemics, *Democratic Theory*, 7:2, 124–33.

Prainsack, B., and Buyx, A. (2011), *Solidarity: Reflections on an Emerging Concept in Bioethics*, Nuffield Council on Bioethics.

Prainsack, B., and Buyx, A. (2017), *Solidarity in Biomedicine and Beyond*, Cambridge University Press.

Prainsack, B., Kittel, B., Kritzinger, S., and Boomgaarden, H. (2020), The Coronation of Austria: Part 11, Blog post on *Medium*. Available at: https://bprainsack.medium.com/the-coronation-of-austria-part-11-204332e202df.

Puska, P. (2007), Health in All Policies, *European Journal of Public Health*, 17:4, 328.

Rasmussen, S. A., Khoury, M. J., and Del Rio, C. (2020), Precision Public Health as a Key Tool in the Covid-19 Response, *JAMA*, 324:10, 933–4.

Self, P. (1993), *Government by the Market? The Politics of Public Choice*, Macmillan.

United Nations Development Programme (2019), *Human Development Report 2019: Beyond Income, beyond Averages, beyond Today: Inequalities in Human Development in the 21st Century*. Available at: http://hdr.undp.org/en/2019-report/download.

Wagenaar, H. and Wenninger, F. (2020). Deliberative policy analysis, interconnectedness and institutional design: lessons from "Red Vienna", *Policy Studies*, 41(4): 411–37.

Wagenaar, H., and Prainsack B. (2021), *The Pandemic Within: Policy Making for a Better Society*, Policy Press.

Wilson, J. Q. (1989), *Bureaucracy. What Government Agencies Do and Why They Do It*, Basic Books.

Index

Note: Tables and figures are indicated by an italic "*t*" and "*f*" following the page number.

#WeAreNotWaiting 128, 208
1 + Million Genomes 32

access to medicines *see* health access
    movements
activism, healthcare 4–5
    collective good 5–7, 14–16, 17, 22–3
    continuum 15
    defined 2, 48
    see also data activism; evidence-based;
        invited activism; patient activism
ACT UP 63, 70
advocacy groups
    cervical cancer 140–2, 158–60
    healthcare context 146–7
    patient activism 144–6
    practices 147–58
    role 142–4
AFM-Téléthon 57, 59, 64–5, 75–6,
    77–8, 79
Africa, precision medicine and genomics
    initiatives 32, 40
agency, patient 201
    diabetes 208–9, 214–17
AIDS *see* HIV/AIDS
AKU Society UK 58–9, 65, 71–5, 79
Alcoholics Anonymous 61
alkaptonuria 58–9, 65, 71–5
All of Us Research Program 12, 31–2, 34,
    44, 46
Alston, Philip 134
altruism
    corporate 180
    precision medicine and genomics
        initiatives 35, 41
Apple 8, 127
Applegate, Christina 173
Attention Deficit Hyperactivity
    Disorder 63

Australia
    breast cancer 173
    cervical cancer screening policies 155,
        156–7, 161n3
Austria
    Covid-19 pandemic 224–5, 230
    Red Vienna 229
autonomy, patient
    cardiomyopathy 214
    diabetes 209
AveXis 75

Banting, Frederick 218n2
Barry, Michael 87
Bates, Katy 173
"big data" 12–13, 232
"Big Pharma"
    healthcare markets 55–6, 81n4
    precision medicine 12
    social media 108, 109, 110
"Big Tech" 12, 13, 132
Biogen 76, 92
biological citizenship 203
    breast cancer movement 166, 183, 188–9,
        190, 192
Brazil, healthcare markets 56
breast cancer
    experiential knowledge 63
    high-profile nature of 168–9
    public attention and fundraising 161n5
    social movements 20–1, 165–70, 187–92
        dramatis personae 187*t*
        environmental movement and
            cancerogenic pollutant 179–80,
            188–92
        epidemiological narrative and the
            previvor 171–7, 188–91
        feminist narrative and the empowered
            collective 183–92

238 INDEX

breast cancer (*cont.*)
    peri- and post-illness 169–70, 180–92
    pink ribbon narrative and the
        survivor 181–4, 188–92
    pre-illness 169, 170–80, 188–92
Breast Cancer Action 178
   "Think Before You Pink" campaign 179,
    180
Breast Cancer Fund 179
Breast Cancer Research Stamp 182–3
Buchanan, James 227

Campaign for Safe Cosmetics 179
Campos, Hugo 214, 215
Canada, breast cancer 173
cancer 168–9
   datafication 33–4, 119–20, 125, 129, 130
   see also breast cancer; cervical cancer
       screening policies; gynecological
       cancers; lung cancer; ovarian cancer
cancerogenic pollutant narrative, breast
    cancer 177–80, 189, 192
cardiomyopathy
   data activism 214
   experiential knowledge 65
Cerezyme® 76
cervical cancer screening policies 140–2,
    158–60
   advocacy groups
     practices 147–58
     role 142–4
   healthcare context 146–7
   patient activism 144–6
China 134
chronic illnesses
   datafication 119, 129–30
   experiential knowledge 60–1, 68
   see also diabetes
citizen science 202–3
Clinton, Hillary 182
collaborative governance, Denmark 117,
    119, 120, 128–9, 132–4
collective good 1
   Covid-19 pandemic 9–10, 14–16, 22, 229,
    231–2
   datafication 12–13
   healthcare activism 5–7, 14–16, 17, 22–3
   healthcare market 2–4, 8–11, 14–16, 18, 19
   individual freedom versus 14

and inequality 229
marginal voices 22
medical science 11–13
multiple voices 9–11
patient activism 10–11, 20, 141, 160
precision medicine 12–13, 15–16
prevention paradigm 14
theoretical frameworks 7–9
see also public goods
common good 6
   see also collective good
Compassionate Use patient programs 11
compliance, patient 198–201, 214, 216
confidentiality issues 131
   see also privacy issues
consumerism
   breast cancer, survivor narrative 183, 191–2
   diabetes 215–16
   marketization 13, 88
   precision medicine 13, 14
   US healthcare 211
continuous glucose monitors (CGMs) 128,
    199, 205–9
Conway, Paul 210–11
Copenhagen Catalogue 132
Copenhagen Letter 132
cost evaluation 56, 58–9, 69, 73–5, 79–80
Covid-19 1
   anti-vaccination activists 15, 16
   collective good 9–10, 14–16, 22, 229, 231–2
   datafication 132
   healthcare markets 2, 3–4, 9
   healthcare context 146–7
   impact 224–32
   medication 10
   personal and protective equipment 2, 3–4,
    226
   skeptics 15, 16
   state–civil social relationship 22
   vaccine 2, 4, 6, 9–10, 226, 228
credentialized knowledge, cervical cancer
    screening policies 142, 159–60
   advocacy groups' practices 148–58
   patient activism 144
cystic fibrosis (CF) 86–7, 91–2, 93–4,
    96–106
Cytodiagnostics in Sweden 158

DanAge 122
Danish Business Authorities 132

Danish Consumer Council 122
data activism 119
  cardiomyopathy patients 214
  Denmark 118, 131–2
  diabetes patients 206–8
data-driven medicine 12, 15
  see also datafication; precision medicine
datafication 12, 19–20, 116–18, 133–5, 232
  collective good 12–13
  opposition 119, 131–2
  patient activism 118–20, 127–31
  patient voices 116, 118, 126–7, 130
  power struggles 118–22
  right to data 122–5
Data for Good 131
data protection 35, 36
deaf people
  empowerment 202
  experiential knowledge 62
deliberative democracy 9
Denmark
  andels movement 120
  datafication 19–20, 116–35
  PRO initiative 126–7
  Sundhed.dk 122–5, 127, 129
  welfare state development 120–1
DevelopAKUre 72
development of drugs, and patient
      organizations 58–60, 68–72, 79
deviant activism 15
Dexcom 207
diabetes
  datafication 119, 128–9
  experiential knowledge 60
  patient empowerment 199–200, 203–4
  patient-designed devices 128–9, 198–9,
    205–10, 212–17
disabled people 62, 63, 68
DIY Pancreas System 208
Duchenne muscular dystrophy 64

Earthjustice 178–9
employers, and datafication 123, 124
empowered collective narrative, breast
    cancer 183–7
empowerment *see* patient empowerment
engagement, patient 200, 201, 203, 210–11
  diabetes 199, 204, 213–15
environmental diseases 63

environmental movement and breast
    cancer 177–80, 188–92
epidemiological narrative, breast
    cancer 171–7
Estée Lauder, Breast Cancer Awareness
    range 182
European Medicines Agency 72, 93
European Union (EU)
  Covid-19 pandemic 3, 4
  Directive on Orphan Medicinal
    Products 58, 66, 76
  healthcare markets 8, 59, 77
  orphan drugs 86, 105
EURORDIS 58, 59, 66–7, 77, 79
  Round Table of Companies (ERTC) 58, 59,
    82n12
Evangelista, Linda 182, 186
evidence-based activism 20
  cervical cancer screening policies 142,
    159–60
    advocacy groups' practices 147–58
    patient activism 144–5
  datafication 116, 118, 130
  experiential knowledge 60, 64–8
  healthcare markets 58–9, 69, 71,
    77, 79–80
exit 28, 36
  precision medicine and genomics
    initiatives 29–30, 37–46, 48, 50
experiential knowledge 144–5
  cervical cancer screening policies 141,
    161n6
  healthcare markets 71, 72
  patient organizations, dynamics and
    epistemic role of 60–9

Facebook *see* social media
feminist narrative, breast cancer 179,
    180–1, 183–92
Fire in the Blood 56
Fitbit 127
FORCE 171–2, 175
France
  Centre national de la recherche
    scientifique 75
  experiential knowledge 64–5
  healthcare markets 57, 59, 75–6, 77–8
  Observatoire économique du medicament
    orphelin 77–8

240 INDEX

France (*cont.*)
  public ownership of pharmaceutical
    industry 24n9
fundraising
  breast cancer 161n5, 168, 180, 181–3, 190
  rare diseases 64, 86, 93, 104–6

Gaucher disease 76
Généthon 75
genetic data, sharing 28–30, 32–3
  benefits 33–4, 35–6
  costs 34–6
  exit, opt-out, and voice 37–42
  invited activism 47–50
  participatory medicine 42–7
genetic discrimination 35
genetic disease patients 33–4, 35–6, 46–7
Genome Asia 100K 32
Genomics England 31–2, 34, 44–7
genomics initiatives 11–12, 13
  exit, opt-out, and voice 36–42
  genetic data, sharing 32–6
  invited activism 28–31, 47–50
  participatory medicine 42–7
  see also precision medicine
Genzyme 76
Ghebreyesus, Tedros Adhanom 6
Gilead 10
GitHub 208, 218n6
Google 8, 127
Gulf War Syndrome 63
Guterres, Antonio 6
Gynae Cancer Group (GCG) 140–2, 158–60
  healthcare context 146–7
  patient activism 144–6
  practices 147–58
  role 143, 144
gynecological cancers 20, 146–7, 149
  see also cervical cancer screening policies;
    ovarian cancer

Hammid, Hella 186
Hanneman, Chris 208
Harris, Simon 99, 112n18
Havasupai Indians 40
Hawaii University 71
health access movements 4, 17, 29
  datafication 128
  healthcare markets 59, 77, 79

healthcare activism *see* activism, healthcare
healthcare markets *see* markets, healthcare
health data, sharing 123–4
health management organizations 81n2
health professionals, and
    datafication 123–5
health social movements 4–5
  breast cancer 165–8, 169–70
    dramatis personae 187t
    environmental movement and
      cancerogenic pollutant 179–80,
      188–92
    epidemiological narrative and the
      previvor 171–7, 188–91
    feminist narrative and the empowered
      collective 183–92
    peri- and post-illness 169–70, 180–92
    pink ribbon narrative and the
      survivor 181–4, 188–92
    pre-illness 169, 170–80, 188–92
  datafication 118
  experiential knowledge 62–3
health technology assessments
    (HTAs) 112n16
  Denmark 116
  Ireland 95–6
heart rehabilitation patients 126
Herceptin 33–4
HIV/AIDS
  patient activism 14, 17, 128, 144
    experiential knowledge 63
    and feminist cancer activism 183–4, 185
    healthcare markets 56, 70
  patient empowerment 202
Human Genome Project 175
human papillomavirus (HPV) screening
    policies 140–2, 158–9, 161nn4, 9
  advocacy groups
    practices 148–58
    role 143–4
  patient activism 145, 146
human right, health as 4
hybrid forums 9, 118
hypertrophic cardiomyopathy 214

implanted pacemakers 214, 215
inequalities
  breast cancer movement 185, 187, 188
  cervical cancer screening policies 151–4

and the collective good 229
compliance dependency on 200
datafication 127
diabetes technologies, access to 210
precision medicine 41
and social unrest 225
reducing 231
innovation *see* research and development
Instagram *see* social media
insulin
    patent 218n2
    price 210, 215
    pumps 128, 205–9, 213
insurance companies
    datafication 124
    healthcare markets 81n2
intellectual property rights 9, 228–9
    healthcare markets 56, 57, 69
    see also patents
invited activism 15, 17, 141
    datafication 118, 126–7
    defined 29
    evidence-based activism 144
    precision medicine and genomics
        initiatives 28–31, 47–50
Ireland
    drug reimbursement assessment
        process 95f, 95–6
    Health Act (2013) and amendment (Bill 33,
        2018) 87, 96, 109–10
    Health Information and Quality Authority
        (HIQA) 96
    Health (Pricing and Supply of Medical
        Goods) Act (2013) 86
    Health Service Executive (HSE) 86, 95–6,
        108
        Orkambi 86–7, 93, 97, 99–101
        Spinraza 87, 93, 101
    National Centre for Pharmacoeconomics
        (NCPE) 19, 86–7, 95–6, 108
        Orkambi 87, 92, 99
        Spinraza 87, 93, 101
    patient activism
        healthcare markets 81n4
        orphan drugs 86–7, 91–111

Jolie, Angelina 173–5

Kushner, Rose, *Breast Cancer* 187

laboratory results, and datafication 124–5
Lacks, Henrietta 40
Leibrand, Scott 208
Lewis, Dana 208, 213
LGBTQ+ community 62, 185
Look, Howard 213
Loop 209
Lorde, André, *The Cancer Journals* 187
loyalty 28
    precision medicine and genomics
        initiatives 39, 40–3
lung cancer 169

Madelin, Robert 67
Madsen-Mygdal, Thomas 131–2
marketization 2–3, 87–8
    collective good 10
    consumerism 13, 88
markets, healthcare 2–4
    collective good 2–4, 8–11, 14–16, 18, 19
    Covid-19 pandemic 225–32
    data-driven medicine 12
    healthcare activism 17
    patient activism 55–9, 68–81
        social media, advocacy role 87–91,
            109, 111
    war on disease 18
Matuschka 185–6
medical science, and the collective good 11
Medtronic 206, 207
Metzger, Deena 186
MISFIRES and Market Innovation
    project 5, 31
moral issues
    collective good 5, 7, 8, 9, 16
    Compassionate Use patient programs 11
    Covid-19 pandemic 224–5, 229, 231, 232
    datafication 117, 134
    healthcare activism 15, 16, 23
    healthcare market 3–4, 11, 13, 15
    health risk management, and breast
        cancer 191
    medical science 11
    patient activism, and social media 89–90,
        107
    rare disease patient organizations 80–1
    solidarity 224–5
multiple sclerosis 60
muscular dystrophy 64

242 INDEX

mutual aid movement 61, 64
  criticisms of 62
myopathy 57, 64–5

neoliberalism
  criticisms 12
  marketization 2, 10, 11
  patient empowerment 21
  precision medicine 13
  prevention paradigm 14
  self-management 21
New Public Management 228
Newton-John, Olivia 173
Nightscout 208
nitisinone 58–9, 71–3, 75
non-compliance, patient 198–201, 214, 216
Novartis 75

Obama, Barack 12
obesity 232
O'Day, Daniel 10
Ogliastra people 40
OmniPod 205
Open Android 209
Open APS 208, 209
open source movement 218n2
  diabetes technologies 198, 199, 204,
    209–10, 212–16
opting out 36–7
  of sharing genetic data 36, 37–40, 42, 45,
    47, 50
orders of worth framework 7–8, 23n4
Orkambi 19, 86–7, 91–2, 93–4, 96–106
  timeline of campaign highlights 98f
  timeline of political highlights 100f
  tweet categories 94f, 104f
orphan drugs
  healthcare markets 57–9, 74, 75–80
  social media 86–7, 91–111
Osbourne, Sharon 173
ovarian cancer 147, 168
  CA125 blood test 153
  risk of 171, 174

pacemakers 214, 215
Pap smear policies 140, 142, 159, 161nn4, 9
  advocacy groups
    practices 147–8, 150, 152, 154–8
    role 142–4

participant involvement, precision
    medicine and genomics
    initiatives 30, 45–50
participatory medicine, precision medicine
    and genomics initiatives 30–1,
    42–50
participatory turn 31, 37, 43
patents
  Covid-19 vaccine 9
  healthcare markets 3, 56, 71, 75
  insulin 218n2
patient activism 4
  breast cancer 20–1
  cervical cancer screening policies 140–2,
    144–6, 158–60
    advocacy groups' practices 147–58
    advocacy groups' role 142–4
    healthcare context 146–7
  collective good 10–11, 20, 141, 160
  datafication 118–20, 125, 127–31
  diabetes 199–200, 203–4
    patient-designed devices 198–9,
      205–10, 212–17
  dynamics and epistemic role of patient
    organizations 59–69
  empowerment 202
  gynecological cancer 20
  healthcare markets 55–9, 68–81, 87–91,
    109, 111
  marginal voices 21–2
  social media 19, 86–111
  war on disease 18
patient agency 201
  diabetes 208–9, 214–17
patient autonomy
  cardiomyopathy 214
  diabetes 209
patient compliance/non-
    compliance 198–201, 214, 216
Patient Data Association
    (Patientdataforeningen,
    Denmark) 131, 132
patient empowerment 21, 200–3
  breast cancer 191
    feminist narrative 184–5
    previvor narrative 172, 174–5, 176
  datafication 19–20, 117–20, 122–5, 127,
    131
  diabetes 198–9, 203–4

INDEX   243

patient-designed devices 21, 198–9, 205–10, 212–17
experiential knowledge 63, 65
precision medicine and genomics initiatives 34, 39
prevention paradigm 14
social media 89
US Food and Drug Administration 201, 203, 204, 210–14
patient engagement 200, 201, 203, 210–11
diabetes 199, 204, 213–15
patient involvement, precision medicine and genomics initiatives 29–31, 45–50
patient-reported outcomes (PRO)
datafication 126–7, 130
US 211
personalized medicine 11–12, 13, 32
see also precision medicine
pink ribbon narrative, breast cancer 179, 180, 181–3, 191
Plant, Barry 91
precision medicine 12
access dynamics 17–18
collective good 12–13, 15–16
defined 32, 33
exit, opt-out, and voice 37–9, 41
genetic data, sharing 32–4
invited activism 28–31, 47–50
participatory medicine 43–6
see also genomics initiatives; personalized medicine
prevention paradigm 14
previvor narrative, breast cancer 171–7, 188–91
price of medications 18–19
Compassionate Use patient programs 11
healthcare markets 55–9, 69, 71, 74, 75–81
insulin 210, 215
remdesivir 10
social media 86–7, 92–111
privacy issues
datafication 124, 125, 131, 134
genetic data, sharing 35, 36
public choice economics 227–8
public goods 6, 227
precision medicine and genomics initiatives 41–2, 43, 50
see also collective good

public involvement, precision medicine and genomics initiatives 29–31, 45–50
public–private partnerships 12–13
PXE International 71

Rackleyft, Nate 208–9
rare disease patients
activism 144
dynamics and epistemic role of patient organizations 59–60, 63, 64–9
healthcare markets 57–9, 69, 71–80
social media 86–8, 91–111
genetic data, sharing 33
Redgrave, Lynn 173
Red Vienna 229
remdesivir 10
research and development (R&D)
breast cancer 168–9, 177, 181, 182–3, 190
collective good 9
datafication 119, 121, 128–9
opposition to 131–2
diabetes 217
diagnostic companies 144
gynecological cancers 147
healthcare markets 2, 58, 69–72, 75, 77, 79–80
HIV/AIDS 144
market competition 8
participatory design in clinical research 202–3
patient empowerment in the US 210, 211
patient organizations, dynamics and epistemic role of 59, 63–8
precision medicine and genomics initiatives 29–45, 49–50
public–private partnerships 13
public sector 228–30
social media 89, 111
Revlon 179
right to data 122–5
rights-based conception of healthcare 4, 121
Roche Diagnostics 143, 144

Schwamb, Pete 208
Scibilia, Renza 198–9, 200, 215, 217
science, medical, and the collective good 11
self-help movement 61, 64
criticisms of 62

244 INDEX

Sigler, Holli, *Breast Cancer Journal* 186
SMAIrelandCom 93–4, 101, 103–6
  tweet categories 95f, 104f
Sobi 72
social media
  breast cancer movement 175–6, 182
  cervical cancer screening policies 146,
    151–2, 154, 156–8
  datafication 123, 128, 131
  diabetes 128, 204, 208
  healthcare market advocacy 87–91
  Ireland's pricing of orphan drugs 86–7,
    93–4, 94f, 95f, 96–111
  patient activism 19
  political polarization 230
  roles
    challenging powerful actors 108, 109f,
      110
    enrollment of new actors 106–7, 109f,
      110
    extension of the community 109f,
      109, 110
    mobilization of actors offline 107–8,
      109f, 110
    renegotiation of value
      definitions 109f, 109–10
social movements *see* health social
  movements
solidarity 224–5, 231
Solomon, Barbara 185
Sontag, Susan, *Illness as Metaphor* 187
South Africa, healthcare markets 56
Spain, marketization of healthcare 88
Spence, Jo, "Marked Up for
  Amputation" 186
spinal muscular atrophy (SMA) 64–5,
  75–6, 87, 92–4, 101–7
Spinraza 19, 76, 87, 92–4, 101–7, 109
  timeline of campaign and political
    highlights 102f
  tweet categories 95f, 104f
Steno Diabetes Center Copenhagen
  (SDCC) 128–9
Sundhed.dk 122–5, 127, 129
surveillance capitalism 121, 132, 134–5
survivor narrative, breast cancer 181–4,
  188–92
Sveriges Cytodiagnostiker 158

Sweden
  cervical cancer screening policies 140–2,
    158–60
    advocacy groups' practices 147–58
    advocacy groups' role 143, 144
    healthcare context 146–7
    patient activism 144–6
    "Saving Women's Lives" 148–50
    National Board of Health and Welfare
      (NBHW) 140, 146, 148–58, 161n9
Swedish Cancer Registry 157, 158
Swedish Cancer Society 154

Techfestival 131–2
Thatcher, Margaret 227
therapeutic development, and patient
  organizations 58–60, 68–72, 79
Three Million African Genomes 32
tolerated activism 15
Trastuzumab 33–4
Twitter *see* social media
type 1 diabetes (T1D) 199–200, 203–4
  patient-designed devices 21, 198–9,
    205–10, 212–17

United Kingdom
  alkaptonuria 73–5
  breast cancer 169, 173, 182
  Department of Health 74
  experiential knowledge 65
  Genomics England 31–2, 34, 44–7
  healthcare markets 58–9, 71–5, 88
  National Health Service (NHS) 73–4
  National Institute for Health and Care
    Excellence (NICE) 74–5, 81n8
  off-label law 73
  Universal Basic Services (UBS) 225–6,
    233n2
United States
  21st Century Cures Act (2016) 201, 211
  "All of Us" initiative 12, 31–2, 34,
    44, 46
  breast cancer 168, 179, 202
  cervical cancer screening policies 143–4,
    150, 158, 161n3
  Covid-19 pandemic 226
  datafication 134
  diabetes 199, 210, 215

Food and Drug Administration (FDA)
  cancerogenic food flavor
    chemicals 179
  Centers for Device and Radiological
    Health (CDRH) 210, 211, 212
  diabetes devices 128, 205, 207, 213,
    214
  HPV test 143
  orphan drugs 75, 77, 92
  patient empowerment 201, 203, 204,
    210–14
  Patient Engagement Advisory
    Committee (PEAC) 210–11
healthcare markets 81n2
healthcare system 204
HIV/AIDS patient activism 202
Meaningful Use policy 201
National Cancer Institute 168
non-compliance 214
Orphan Drug Act (1983) 76, 77, 88
self-help movement 61
spinal muscular atrophy 92
Universal Basic Services (UBS) 225–6,
    233n2

Vertex Pharmaceuticals 92, 97, 99–101
voice 28, 31, 36
  datafication 116, 118, 126–7, 130
  Food and Drug Administration 211
  marginal voices 21–2
  precision medicine and genomics
    initiatives 29–30, 37–40, 41–50

war on disease 18
  experiential knowledge 60, 63–8
  healthcare markets 58, 69–70, 75, 79–80
#WeAreNotWaiting 128, 208
Wellcome Trust Sanger Institute 40
West, Ben 207, 208, 213
World Health Organization (WHO) 4
World Trade Organization (WTO) 9
worth, orders of 7–8, 23n4

YesOrkambi 93–4, 96–106
  timeline of campaign highlights 98*f*
  timeline of political highlights 100*f*
  tweet categories 94*f*, 104*f*

Zolgensma 75–6